Six Weeks to Sleeveless and Sexy

"We learn by attraction. Just look at JJ Virgin and you will want what she has. This book teaches you how to get it."

—Suzanne Somers

"JJ is my personal nutrition coach and has worked with me on many of the lifestyle recommendations that she will take you through in this book. She is the master at creating simple action steps that you can easily integrate into your life to create new healthy habits that will make a major change to your body and your health."

—Jack Canfield, coauthor of *The Success Principles* and the Chicken Soup for the Soul series

"I have worked with JJ over the years with my patients and consulted with her on my personal health. She is the master at integrating nutrition, exercise and health to create beautiful outcomes. Follow the plan. JJ's program works!"

—Andrew P. Ordon, MD, FACS, cohost of *The Doctors*

"Getting lean, strong and healthy is JJ Virgin's mission and she does it fabulously in this easy to read yet very comprehensive book. If you're looking for a blueprint to get your arms sleeveless and sexy and want to get it done fast, you've found your book! The bonus is the rest of your body will do the same! You can't help but LOVE this book."

—Leanne Ely, *New York Times* bestselling author of *Saving Dinner*

"JJ Virgin is a national treasure when it comes to nutrition and fitness, but she also knows how to motivate and inspire. Finally, a health book that's based on sound science. If you want that sexy, sleek and toned look, look no further than this book!"

—Jonny Bowden, PhD, CNS, bestselling author of
The 150 Healthiest Foods on Earth and
The Most Effective Ways to Live Longer

"JJ has been a consultant to Amen Clinics, Inc. and I highly value her work. This book will help you quickly have a better body and even a better brain!"

—Daniel G. Amen, MD, *New York Times* bestselling author
of *Change Your Brain, Change Your Life*; *Magnificent Mind at Any Age*; and *Change Your Brain, Change Your Body*

"I have been working with JJ Virgin for years with wonderful and balanced results. Her programs are tried and true. *Six Weeks to Sleeveless and Sexy* is a must have, a must read. Jam-packed with easy to follow steps for a successful and healthy body and life, JJ brings it home in this inspiring guide."

—Carré Otis, Director of The Network Model Community

"JJ Virgin is the real deal! In a charming, user-friendly style, she delivers clear and accurate guidance for weight loss and fitness. And she walks her talk: she is a perfect example of what she teaches."

—Hyla Cass, MD, author of *8 Weeks to Vibrant Health*

Six Weeks to Sleeveless and Sexy

The 5-Step Plan to Sleek, Strong, and Sculpted Arms

JJ Virgin, PhD, CNS

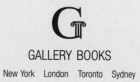

GALLERY BOOKS

New York   London   Toronto   Sydney

G

Gallery Books
A Division of Simon & Schuster, Inc.
1230 Avenue of the Americas
New York, NY 10020

First Gallery Books trade paperback edition May 2010

GALLERY BOOKS and colophon are trademarks of Simon & Schuster, Inc.

Photography by Lesley Bohm

Makeup and Styling by Tamara Gold

For information about special discounts for bulk purchases,
please contact Simon & Schuster Special Sales at
1-866-506-1949 or business@simonandschuster.com.

The Simon & Schuster Speakers Bureau can bring authors to your live event.
For more information or to book an event contact the Simon & Schuster Speakers Bureau
at 1-866-248-3049 or visit our website at www.simonspeakers.com.

Designed by Ruth Lee-Mui

Manufactured in the United States of America

3   5   7   9   10   8   6   4

Library of Congress Cataloging-in-Publication Data

Virgin, J J.
Six weeks to sleeveless and sexy : the 5-step plan to sleek, strong and sculpted arms / JJ Virgin.
    p.   cm.
1. Arm exercises.   2. Shoulder exercises.   3. Exercise for women.   I. Title.
GV508.V57   2010
613.71082—dc22   2010011514

ISBN 978-1-4391-8934-4
ISBN 978-1-4391-9043-2 (ebook)

Note to Readers

This publication contains the opinions and ideas of its author. It is intended to provide helpful and informative material on the subjects addressed in the publication. It is sold with the understanding that the author and publisher are not engaged in rendering medical, health, or any other kind of personal professional services in the book. The reader should consult his or her medical, health, or other competent professional before engaging in any exercise or diet program or adopting any of the suggestions in this book or drawing inferences from it.

In addition, the author occasionally recommends certain products, services, or websites in the book and its resources section. The recommendations are based on the author's high regard for the product/service mentioned. In the case of Metabolic Maintenance, X-iser, Tanita, Zeo, Emergen-C, and Vital Choice, the author has a professional relationship with or interest in the product/service, and www.jjvirgin.com is her own website store; the author does not have any affiliation with the other products/services recommended.

The author and publisher specifically disclaim all responsibility for any liability, loss, or risk, personal or otherwise, which is incurred as a consequence, directly or indirectly, of the use and application of any of the contents of this book.

This book is dedicated to all of the women who shared their stories, struggles, and pain with me. You inspired me to get my program out there. The confidence you will gain through fully committing to this program will empower all areas of your life.

Contents

Six Weeks to Sleeveless and Sexy

Introduction

The *Dr. Phil* episode was known as "Fat Brides."

First, a disclaimer: I didn't name the show, but there I was on a soundstage on the Paramount lot, an expert in a sea of emotionally ravaged brides, who looked as though they were on the verge of a collective nervous breakdown. Those ladies had "issues" that were more earth-shattering than wilted flowers, a mother-in-law from Hell, or a wayward groom nationally exposed on *Cheaters*.

They were facing the ultimate premarital meltdown: arm fat.

Some women face that dilemma *every single day*.

As one of my friends who recently got hitched told me, "I didn't give a damn about the cake or those personal vows. About ninety percent of wedding dresses now are sleeveless, and

I wanted to weep while standing in the bridal store." After her grandmother and mother convinced her to throw caution (not to mention troubled triceps) to the wind, she plunked down her credit card on a Vera Wang number that turned her never-before-seen-in-public upper arms into a focal point. Later, she regrettably thought they looked like two big clubs Fred Flintstone might have carried around to beat on dinosaurs.

But I digress.

I was the episode guest guru who was there to help the brides get slim and sleek for their special day. And I brought skin calipers to measure their "problem areas." As prearranged with the producers, I grabbed one of the brides, pinched her fat in the most professional, nonjudgmental way possible on national television, and asked, "Are you planning to go sleeveless?"

She burst into tears on the spot.

Believe me when I tell you I felt her pain. I wasn't trying to be a meanie-poo. But I wanted to save her from years of staring at her gorgeous, professionally shot wedding photos and forgetting about the following: her love, her man, her vows, her future.

No, she would just be gazing at those photos in that damn sleeveless nightmare thinking, Why the hell didn't I cover them up with thick Irish lace that went past my wrists? I hate Vera Wang, I hate her. Die, Vera, die!

Yes, women are emotionally distraught over their arms, and that is about to end with this book.

Arms Are the New Accessory

Forget the Gucci purse and the pearl-rimmed Chanel sunglasses. Diamond hoop earrings are nice, as is a healthy collection of Manolo Blahniks. You know what? I'd trade in all of the above for the one accessory that goes with everything and never goes out of style: sleek, strong, and sculpted arms.

My name is JJ Virgin, and I love my arms. Please don't hate me for saying that to you. I know it's almost illegal to say those words aloud without serving time in some Jenny Craig prison, but I will say it again . . . and again: *I love my arms.* They're strong, lean, muscular, and sculpted. They look good in the cheapest $5 tank top from Target or a $5,000 sparkling designer gown. Even on the days when I pile my hair up in a big ponytail and run out without a hint of makeup, women rush up to me and say, "I'm sorry, but I have to ask you: where did you get those arms?"

The truth is, you can't really buy them from some plastic surgeon nor sweat them off with the latest exercise craze. And great arms aren't just about genetics. My arms look this way because of science and an understanding of how the body works, what to eat, how to most effectively exercise, and how to live. With this knowledge, you too can sculpt yourself from within without spending a lot of money or time on the process.

First, a few introductions are in order.

I'm a celebrity health and nutrition expert with twenty-five years of experience in the health and fitness industry. I have a PhD in holistic nutrition and have attended six different graduate and doctoral programs, including biomechanics at California State University, Northridge, sports medicine at University of Miami, doctoral-level courses in exercise physiology, nutrition, and aging at USC, and nutrition at University of Bridgeport. I am currently in a master's program in nutritional and metabolic medicine at the University of South Florida School of Medicine.

That's why I know so much about sculpting arms; I follow the science. I also know there is no hiding them and you shouldn't have to put them under the equivalent of a quilt each time you leave the house.

If you follow my six-week Sleeveless and Sexy Program, you will be like Diane Keaton in the movie *Something's Gotta Give*. Remember when Jack Nicholson was kissing her in bed and suddenly she asked him to cut off the thick white turtleneck that covered her entire upper body? As the scissors sliced through the material and the fresh air hit her skin, she could only sigh in gratitude because she felt something money couldn't buy.

Freedom.

In six weeks, you will be free to flaunt your arms in public. Fresh air will touch skin that perhaps hasn't felt a breeze in the last decade. If you live in a cold-weather climate, please use caution because this will feel so good that you might opt to wear tank tops even when it's ten degrees below outside. You will also rush out to buy that wonderful strappy little black dress and wear it with confidence and pride.

You will finally have the right to bare arms—and feel proud of your arms that are bare.

Arms: A Historical Perspective

We're not the only generation that has struggled with the right to bare arms. My grandmother was a thin woman, but she had an odd situation going on up top: her arm fat draped down like two veils. I remember playfully flapping her arm veils around, and they would swing to and fro. Of course, she didn't really mind because she was a granny and strappy tank tops weren't exactly on her list of must-have fashion items.

When I first worked as a personal trainer some twenty-five years ago, women didn't even use hand weights. I had to sneak them in during aerobics classes. I would also have them do push-ups and they would protest, "That's a guy's exercise. I'm going to bulk up and look like a football player." (Absolutely untrue, but more on that later.) I would even take some of my clients to Gold's Gym in Venice, California, and they would shriek, "I don't want to look like those he-man body builders!" These were women who weighed *140 pounds*. There was no chance of their bulking up unless they started doing mass doses of steroids.

Now women understand exercise a bit better, and they want that lean, firm, muscular look. They also know that they need muscles because that sort of toning is sexy and holds everything in tighter. Just look at any of the major female stars of our day, including Halle Berry, Kelly Ripa, Angela Bassett, Jennifer Lopez, and Blake Lively. Their arms are for public consumption in those gorgeous designer gowns.

Muscles are also a metaphor for something larger: empowerment. Arms represent strength. They're symbolic of not being the little waify woman who needs a man to lift and carry for her. If you have muscles, you're not weak. Arms say you can handle things. (And what if there's a fire and you need to lower yourself out of a window—could you do it?) It turns out that strong arms are also practical and functional. Who knew?

This brings me to a question I'm asked over and over again: "JJ, how did my arms get so bad?" Well, as with any slippery slope, you slide down bit by bit over time. Suddenly, you're sort of used to that fat on your arms and you just put a few more layers of clothing over them. As you get older and a little heavier (each year), it seems as though the fat just pours into your arms. Most women don't just gain five pounds a year; they may gain ten pounds of fat and lose five pounds of muscle. Your muscles are your metabolic girdle and hold everything in tighter so that you have shape. Muscles keep your metabolism up all day long. When it comes to your muscles, if you don't use them, you lose them.

In a nutshell, *that's* why your arms are getting worse and worse.

Women do want to get in shape. In fact, they spend a good chunk of change talking to trainers and trying chemically based diet "foods." There are many $75-an-hour trainers who tell their female clients that the way to get their entire body in shape is with a daily hourlong power walk. They promise that simply swinging your arms while walking will tone them up.

Tune out that advice.

A steady power walk is simply controlled falling and really doesn't burn much fat or develop muscle. What I advocate is walking for two minutes and then performing a minute all-out "burst" in which you go as fast as you possibly can. When you burst and recover, your body becomes involved in a major metabolic workout that raises your lactic acid levels. The lactic acid "burn" signals that you are raising your growth hormone levels. Now you're burning more fat, building muscle, and staying young.

Women don't burn fat naturally; we're fat storers in order to have and feed our babies. Arms are a common place to store fat. In order to get rid of that fat, you will have to do burst exercise, eat right, and work on the science that will help you achieve results.

One interesting side note is that women aren't described as "apples" and "pears" anymore when it comes to body shapes. Between our stressful lifestyles and our steady diet of refined carbohydrates and artificial foods, most of us have screwed up our metabolisms to the point where we store fat and gain weight like a man. This means we now carry our fat in our stomachs and our arms.

armed and dangerous

When you look good all over, you will look great in jeans and a T-shirt. You don't need fifty of the same drapey black shirts if you're in shape.

How Many Shrugs Can One Woman Own?

It should make everyone feel much better to know that even Julia Roberts has had arm issues. I'm sorry, Pretty Woman, but I remember your Oscar win (congrats!) and how you flew up to the stage hooting and hollering in that gorgeous black velvet vintage couture gown with the white Y-shaped satin. Everything was perfect, from your preternaturally white smile to your stay-put-in-a-tsunami bun. But you had granny arms. Yes, Jules, time to face facts. Your arms had no visible muscle tone and actually looked a little flabby. Hello, weight resistance program!

I actually sat there thinking, Hasn't anyone noticed how her arms look in that dress? And she is Julia Roberts. Come on! How could her stylist hook her up this way?

Many women are reading this and thinking, "You think Julia had bad arms? Julia and I have now bonded. Julia! She's my girl! Put her in a tube top so we can all feel better about ourselves!"

I know a woman who had gastric bypass surgery. She's around five feet five inches and used to weigh 350 pounds. After getting rid of 180 pounds, all she could talk about was her arms and whether they would ever get in shape. It wasn't looking at her new lean legs in a hot skirt or her waistline that was suddenly denting her in. Instead, she said, "I dream of the day when I can buy an actual sundress and not cover it up with five layers of sweaters."

This brings me to a crucial arms topic: stop covering them up and making them sweat under countless layers of shawls and shrugs. You will never melt the fat that way, plus the damn shrugs are expensive and scream, "I have fat arms that are in some sort of *body witness protection program!*" No one looks good in a shrug unless she weighs about 90 pounds and doesn't need the shrug in the first place.

There is not now, nor will there ever be . . . Spanx for arms.

If you read this book and follow my plan, you won't need Spanx, but you will give *thanks* for giving yourself six weeks to freedom.

In forty-two days, you will be sexy, sleeveless, sculpted, and strong.

The JJ Virgin Arms Treaty

Ladies of all shapes and sizes, I hereby propose the following joint resolution as The JJ Virgin Arms Treaty. This treaty is proposed as binding between you and your new fitness and nutrition expert, JJ Virgin.

We hereby resolve to:

- Abolish forever this phrase from your vocabulary: *Do my arms look fat?*
- Stop the madness of wearing cashmere shrugs over sundresses when it's 98 degrees outside.
- Drop the sneaky way you slink into the background of family pictures so your arms don't look bigger than those of the guys in the photo.
- End all the excuses you have for not going to the beach because there is no Spanx for arms.
- Put to rest your resentment of famous actresses with toned arms. In other words, don't be a toned-arm hater.
- Stop staring at your little three-pound baby hand weights and wondering why a thousand bicep curls seem to do absolutely nothing.
- Be part of a movement where women know they have the right to bare arms and bare them proudly in the sunlight and in the

moonlight, thus allowing fresh air to touch skin that hasn't been uncovered or felt a breeze in years.

Talk to your doctor to make sure you're good to go, and then resolve to do the following:

- Follow the nutrition plan in this book exactly as written.
- Do the weight exercises and cardio-blasting exercises exactly as described.
- Make sure you work on getting stress out of your life (as much as possible) and then deploy effective stress-busting techniques.
- Commit to getting seven to nine hours of quality sleep each night.
- Do this program in its entirety—no substitutions and no whining (because it really is so easy that you'll be mad you tried all that other stuff that never worked).

I resolve to:

- Be there with you every step, curl, blast, bite, drink, push, and pull along the way!

Signed: _____ (Reader)

Signed: _____

1. Start 'Em!

No offense to the thinnest waist in the south, Miss Scarlett O'Hara, of *Gone With the Wind* fame, but tomorrow truly is not another day to start your six-week program. You know the drill: tomorrow will become the day after, and then some vague Tuesday when the planets align and the moon is full.

Make a vow with me to schedule your start date right now! Pull out your calendar and choose one day over the next three to begin the program. Circle the start date on the calendar. Unless there's a real emergency, you will not move this date. And just for the record, a sale at Macy's doesn't constitute a true 911 moment. For this program to work, you've got to take it seriously. Think of the start date like an appointment with a doctor or dentist. It may not be a lot of fun, but you respect its importance and the goal of feeling and looking your best.

Perhaps you've canceled on yourself quite a few times over the years when it came to taking care of your body. Of course, your intentions are always honorable. You mean to get started, but then you have to drive the kids to sports practice and there's that extra work project. And how in the world could you miss that two-hour *American Idol* special episode?

The point is, there will *always* be something else you could do instead of focusing on your health and well-being. Once you accept this, it becomes a case of making a formal appointment with yourself. Carve out the time, stamp it as your own, and don't allow *anything* to get in the way of your new goals—short of the house being on fire or a hurricane sweeping down the street. Inform your family that you're checking out for that time to take care of yourself.

No exceptions. No excuses. And once the results begin, you won't ever look back.

An Important Message from Me . . . to You

By reading this book, you're committing to making life changes. You're entrusting me with your valuable time, body, and dreams.

I take this responsibility very seriously. I will give 100 percent back to you. I'm invested in your success. To that end, I will teach you every single tool available to ensure your victory.

My vow: There is not one thing in this book that I'll ask you to do that won't directly contribute to your goal or that I don't actually do myself. Please do every single thing that I ask of you, because skipping even one small step can make all the difference in the world.

My plan has worked for so many people, and failure isn't an option if you truly follow it.

I know you can do it, and I'm right here next to you.

Okay, enough talking. Let's go!

Task One: Clean Out Your Kitchen

Do you want to live in an emotional war zone when it comes to food and cravings? Just wave the white flag and declare peace by kicking the enemy out of your home. Yes, it's time to do a major overhaul of your kitchen by grabbing an XL-sized garbage bag and tossing the foods that are on my "Most Wanted Enemy List."

Now, I realize some of you may think that you don't need to clean out your kitchen, and you're strong and committed enough to the program to peacefully coexist with the temptations that will be in your line of sight every single day. You can handle it!

Maybe you have a family that can't survive without blue cheese salad dressing and large bags of chemically enhanced microwave popcorn in the house. You're going to show those diet killers that you can walk right past them every single day and not even give them a momentary glance. You might even hiss at them.

So there you are, Ms. Willpower, eating that wonderful grilled chicken salad for lunch, but in order to get to the lettuce in your fridge, you have to navigate around a big tub of home-made rice pudding. The beautiful ripe tomatoes on your counter are sharing counter space with the cheese-covered bagels you bought for your son. An innocent walk into the pantry to find some extra-virgin olive oil means facing the open box of mint chocolate Girl Scout cookies that you purchased to support those cute young carb-pushing girls.

Do you really have the kind of willpower to always say no, always make the right call, and always resist?

Hell, no!

Why would you want to put yourself through all the torment, anyway?

Yes, you could *possibly* do it, but then again, you could possibly skydive and live. Are you really going to take that chance with your body?

For me, it's an all-or-nothing proposal, which is why I'm not living, sleeping, or coexisting with the enemy. I'm tossing it out before that box of chocolate calls to me late at night, saying, "JJ,

I'm here. Come to me just for a minute. You miss me. You know you do. Let's talk."

This is a time when you need to practice tough love and just get rid of any foods that will derail your plan, including these culinary culprits: cookies, cakes, pastries, white bread, bagels, doughnuts, chips, dips, creamy dressings, and anything—or should I say everything—that comes in a box and is full of pre-servatives. Say bye-bye to the fake butter sprays, the microwave popcorn, and those sugary "healthy" (I'm rolling my eyes here) yogurts with fruit on the bottom.

Say these words with me: "There is no such thing as a healthy *light* Thousand Island dressing." It's chock-full of chemicals and sugar, which masks the fact that the fat has been taken out.

My eating plan, which I'll explain in the next chapter, is clean and free of chemicals. You will see amazing results when eating real foods that don't wreak havoc on your system. That's why now is the time to get rid of foods that are full of ingredients you can't pronounce.

armed and dangerous

If you can't pronounce it, don't even try it. Just introduce it to Mr. Hefty Bag. It's not real food.

Surprisingly, there are a number of chemically based foods lurking all over your kitchen. For starters, get rid of anything with the word "diet" in it. Diet foods are mostly not food at all but chemistry experiments. In order to take out the sugar or fat, more sugar or fat has to be added, depending on the promise of the food. Foods that are nonfat are usually higher in sugar. There is also a heap of chemicals thrown in to keep them semitasty. Not only are these foods horrendous for your system (and stop you from losing weight as your body goes into shock mode to process the chemicals), but they're not even satisfying. Ever eat a diet "food" and then crave the real thing before you're even finished taking the last chalky bite?

Chuck all diet *anythings* into the trash. This includes the heavily processed, chemically based diet meals from whatever popular and well-advertised diet plan of the week you're following because some celeb says she dropped 50 pounds and now lives in a bikini even when it's ten below outside. We're happy for her, but we don't need the frostbite or the tasteless, freeze-dried, chemically enhanced, crappy diet foods.

So just understand that you will not be having what she's having.

armed and dangerous
If you feel bad about throwing out perfectly good food, put it into a big bag and donate it to your local homeless shelter or food bank.

Foods to Toss

The Obvious Ones

Cookies

Cakes

Doughnuts

Candy

White bread in any form, including bagels, bialys, and muffins
(English and otherwise)

Waffles

High-sugar breakfast cereals

Jellies, including the sugar-free kind

Ice cream and frozen yogurts

Creamy or sugary salad dressings (read the labels!)

Margarine

Ketchup

Vegetable oils, including corn, safflower, and sunflower

The Not-So-Obvious Ones

All sodas, including the diet ones

Energy and cereal bars

Fruit juices—even the ones that are 100 percent natural

Fat-free flavored yogurt

All diet foods, including diet salad dressings and frozen meals

Microwave popcorn

Anything with artificial sweeteners

Processed soy foods

Dried fruits

Jam made with all fruit

Sugar-sweetened peanut butter

Fat-free chips

Replacement foods will be covered in the next chapter. I promise that you won't starve and soon won't even miss the tossed items.

How to Motivate Yourself

Now that your kitchen is free of problems, it's time to get your head equally clear. The first step in that direction is to think about motivation and how you will stay gung ho and committed during not only the next six weeks but for many months and years to come. Let's be honest here. You will need something concrete to really motivate you when times get hard. There will come a day when you have a big fight with your mother on the phone or your boss is really demanding. Maybe the car won't start and your kids are screaming. Suddenly the idea of motivation is out the window and all you want is a Snickers bar.

Or you didn't work out, and suddenly it's eight o'clock on a cold winter night. You're exhausted because it has been such a long day. You figure that it wouldn't be the end of the world if you just skipped one night of exercise. Then you remember that you already skipped another night . . . and another.

How can you keep from derailing your program? You need something that kicks you in the can when times get hard and all you want to say is "&^%$ it!"

Believe me, at some point you will say, "&*^% it, I want that piece of cake." Or "I'm a little too tired to put on my athletic shoes and move." It happens to all of us. But before you pick up a fork and dig into fatty, sugary frosting or write off the gym, I have an idea that's personal kryptonite against program destroyers.

The Power of Projection

I've found one of the best motivators is simply projecting your ideal body. It may seem silly, but really, I want you to do the following "before" and "after" exercise. I promise it will keep you mentally motivated during even the toughest and most challenging moments.

Hit the magazines and find a picture of an actress or athlete you dream of looking like after completing this program. Maybe you love Hilary Swank's strong, sinewy arms. Perhaps your ideal body currently belongs to Halle Berry, Heidi Klum, or our first lady, Michelle Obama. Who it is doesn't matter one bit. The point is to choose someone who makes you stop each time you see her picture and think, *If only . . .*

Now take a picture of your face, roughly the size of the face of the woman in the photo, and paste your head on the celebrity's body. Make several copies of your creation because you will need them. Put one copy smack in the middle of your fridge, and keep another on you at all times, whether in a purse, wallet, or bag. Keep one on your nightstand and one on your bathroom mirror, and one each in your desk at work and your car. Now when you're running around and just want to say, "Forget it, I'm going to grab a slice of pizza for lunch," you can pull out the picture and renew your commitment.

This photo will be your emergency release valve. When you look at it, what you're really asking yourself is: is this really worth it? Is it really worth it to eat that bag of cookies? Is that dried-out coffee store muffin really worth it? Is that tempting breadbasket worth it? Is it worth it to skip the gym to take a nap? Is it worth it to slog through my cardio burst training giving only half an effort? Half an effort will not result in Hilary Swank–ness. Half an effort won't Klum your body. You can't go all Halle

Berry on everyone if you make burger your king or dairy your queen.

This mental photo trick is for every time you even think, Screw it. It will help remind you why you started this program in the first place. Now, before you point the car in the direction of the mall instead of where you work out, ask yourself, "Did my goals change? Did I suddenly wake up this morning and think, 'I don't really want to look that good anymore'?" If the answer is no, then you will stop yourself and not toss in the towel. Yes, you still want to have the body of Ms. Cameron Diaz, and that photo of your head on her body has your attention.

It's completely normal to have days when your motivation lags and you really don't want to exercise or look at another salad. It's perfectly valid to be tired—no, make that exhausted—after trudging through a day during these stressful times. I too have days where I'd rather go to a spa and eat cake—not necessarily in that order—rather than go outside and do my burst training session (more on that in the exercise chapter). The thing that gets me through the cake day is looking at my motivator photo and cementing the idea (again) of why I want to stick with the program.

Keep Your Progress Journal

Keeping a journal is a great way to write down your goals and then monitor your progress. Paste your inspiration photo on the first page. Next, jot down a few reasons why you want to have better arms. In other words, what will toned arms do for your life?

Be specific about what great arms will do for you. What painful experiences will you never have to face again if you get your arms into shape? There are dozens, but for one, you won't have to avoid buying certain clothes. And no one will grab your fatty upper arm and ask if you plan to lose some weight. And guess what? You won't have to sweat under those annoying shrugs on a warm summer evening, nor will you be embarrassed at the gym or think, Why even bother? Even better, you won't dread family vacations or slink away when it's picture time, or hate formal events because all the gorgeous dresses are sleeveless. (Damn those designers!) But best of all, you won't have to spend hours in a mall trying on clothes that hide your arms.

How many years have you suffered from most of the above? How many events have you missed? How many vacations weren't as good as they could have been because you didn't feel confident? And how many excuses have you fabricated to avoid embarrassment?

No, toned arms aren't going to create world peace. But they will create peace of mind for you because suddenly you will be able to walk into a party in a sleeveless dress and not feel self-conscious, and you won't recoil when someone suggests a beach vacation because—oh, the horror of it all—you will have to wear a bathing suit. Maybe you won't have to feel bad at your child's soccer game because it's 100 degrees outside and you dared to wear (*gasp!*) a tank top.

These opening pages of your journal are a wonderful opportunity for you to write down all the benefits and goals of having great arms. Again, on days when your motivation lags, it will be extremely helpful to glance at them and remind yourself why you're working hard. They will help you reach for your dreams again and go for it.

I'm not saying that toned arms will change your life. But I am convinced of one thing: the confidence that comes from feeling good about your arms and, subsequently, your entire body will make all the difference—not only physically but also emotionally.

It's very important and helpful to write down *specific goals*. Let's say your friend is getting married in two months and you're required to wear a sleeveless bridesmaid's dress. Write down that goal, and back it up by adding another paragraph about how you will feel walking around the reception feeling good about your bare arms instead of trying to hide them under some annoying wrap that's trailing in your soup. Or let's say that your husband really wants to go on a romantic trip to Hawaii over the holidays. Your goal could easily be to have great arms to flash in the strappy, figure-hugging sundresses that go so well with anything involving an island.

Special events or other specific goals are wonderful motivators.

I have a client who was in a steamy long-distance relationship in which she saw her significant other only once a month for a long weekend. Yes, she missed him between visits, but it was the best exercise motivator around because she had target dates to look her best and flash her new arms in a slinky little black dress—and an even slinkier one thirty days later.

Goals will keep you going through the dark times when motivation lags. Hurdles will come because life is unpredictable and full of challenges. You just have to be prepared to sail over those hurdles using whatever motivates you best.

armed and dangerous

Wait a second! You didn't do the picture yet and feel that you might just skip that part because it takes too much effort. That picture is not optional. Please do it *now*!

What Else Do I Need to Start?

My program doesn't require a lot of fitness equipment, and what you do need can be purchased very cheaply.

- **Dumbbells.** Invest in some dumbbells, but don't buy those teeny-tiny ones that I joke about making great paperweights for your desk. You will need a range of weights, as some of the exercises use larger muscle groups, which require heavier weights. If you are

Oh, No, My Trainer Is Ticked Off!

It's almost like a dating situation. If you have a personal trainer and then tell him or her that you're about to embark on a new program, he or she will probably drop a 10-pound weight and toss you a hangdog hurt look. It's almost as if you're cheating with another fitness expert! Don't feel guilty or get stuck in the middle. If you showed ten different trainers or nutritionists the same program, each one would have an opinion and tweak the new plan to make it sound an awful lot like their own plan. Experts have a way of wanting to criticize something new because that's their job. We're a verbal group with definite opinions.

You don't really need to work with a trainer when following my program. If you want to, explain that you're doing something new and would like to incorporate it into your workout with the trainer. As for my program, I can vouch for the results all day long. There is a specific and scientific reason for everything you're about to do. Make sure you make this program your priority, and if you still see a trainer, have him or her ensure that you are doing the exercises correctly and pushing up the intensity. Think of your trainer as your accountability partner to help you get the job done.

just starting out, get a pair of 5-, 8-, and 12-pound dumbbells. If you are a regular exerciser, you probably already have a sense of your strength and ability. Your range may start at 8 or 10 pounds and go up as high as 25 pounds! (I have been known to hoist a few 35-pounders here and there, so don't let the high numbers scare you, they will make you sleek and toned, not big and buff.) You will always want to lift the heaviest weights you can safely handle in good form for 8 to 12 repetitions.

Weights are dirt cheap these days, but don't waste your money on those pretty "dumbbells for ladies" that are pink with polka dots and cost three times as much as the basic ones. Your weights just need to weigh what they're supposed to weigh. There is no point in spending big money on something that is purely functional. The ones at Walmart, Kmart, or Target will work just fine! Remember, your weights are not an accessory!

- **A Big Burst-Proof Fitness Ball.** You will use an inflatable fitness ball as your weight bench to do chest presses, along with various other exercises. There are so many great variations of exercises that you can do with a ball. It's important to pay close attention to choosing a ball for your height and inflating it properly based on your needs. (See inflation instructions in chapter 4.)
- **A Bench or Wide Chair without Arms.** You will be using this to do your exercise dips off of. You can use a chair, coffee table, bench, or whatever else you have that works for this purpose.

How to Choose the Right Fitness Ball

Choosing the proper-size ball will ensure that you maximize your workout and maintain good form. There are several ways to determine which size is appropriate for your body. You can use the 90-degree rule: when seated on the ball with your feet flat, your hips and knees should be at or slightly above a 90-degree angle. Or you can use the following table as a general guideline to match your height with an appropriate ball size.

Your Height and Ball Size

4'11" to 5'3": 55 centimeters (about 21 inches) inflated

5'4" to 5'10": 65 centimeters (about 25 inches) inflated

5'11" or taller: 75 centimeters (about 29 inches) inflated

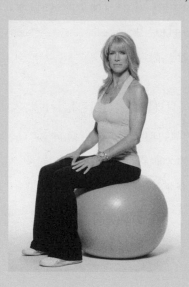

- **An Exercise Mat.** A colorful mat, with your weights lined up neatly in the corner, can be very inviting. You could just throw down a big beach towel on the floor, but I prefer that you invest in an exercise mat and place it in one designated area of your house to do your arm exercises. It helps create an environment for success. It's not your cat's place or where you throw clothes that need dry cleaning.

- **A Good Pair of Workout Shoes.** Don't go crazy thinking you need a new shoe for every different activity. For walking and running, buy a good running shoe. A good cross-trainer will serve all other purposes. I do think that you should invest in high-quality shoes, so this is an area in which to plunk down a little extra cash. Your shoes should serve you for at least six months, and since you will be in them almost every single day, you will want to make sure that they're ultracomfortable and really do fit well.

armed and dangerous

If you haven't purchased a new pair of athletic shoes in the last six months and you wear them almost every day, then toss them. Look at the bottom of shoes that seem iffy. If they look tired and old, it's time to invest in a new pair. Working out in old, worn-down shoes is a great way to get injured.

Optional Equipment

- **A Jump Rope.** It's a cheap option and great for burst training. A jump rope is a handy tool for ladies who travel a lot because you can toss it into a suitcase and use it in your hotel room.

- **An X-iser.** It's my favorite little burst training machine and will travel easily with you. You can use it anywhere and everywhere. This is a totally versatile way to train. Don't buy a cheap imitation. I recommend ordering the one found at www.bursttoblastfat.com that I use with all my private clients. It's so strong that my teen and "tween" boys couldn't demolish it.

Now that you've gathered your equipment, you're just about ready to begin. Make it clear to your family that your workout area is off limits to them. There is nothing worse than reaching for your 5-pound weight and then realizing your son has used it to kill G.I. Joe, and now it's under his bed.

The rule should be: No one enters your workout zone, and no one touches what's in it. *Them's the rules.* And when you're choosing a spot, I prefer that you not set up your workout area in front of the distracting TV. Now, *music* is a great motivator. It's far better to work out to a great pop or rock song than to try to focus while simultaneously watching housewives on Bravo go for each other's throats. And you want to make sure that the music is up-beat and high energy. No offense to Enya, but I'll take Aerosmith anytime during a workout. Michael Bublé might be good for romance, but Michael Jackson is better for working on your triceps. You don't need the sound track from *Yentl* here. The point is to shut off your TV and crank up the tunes because that will tell your brain that it's workout time.

And finally—It's about Your Time Commitment

You made a commitment to yourself by picking up this book and gathering the required equipment. You have your motivation photo at your fingertips. The last piece of the puzzle is making solid time commitments between you—and you—to do your workouts.

When are you going to do the exercises in this book? You can't just say, "Oh, JJ, I'll do them after I put the kids to bed." And I don't want to hear "I like to keep things flexible because I'm a free spirit. Sometimes I'll do them before work, and other times I'll do them before I make dinner."

Leaving the times of your workouts up to fate is a great way to fail. All of us lead busy lives, and it's very easy for time to just run out.

I want you to write in your journal the exact times each

week that you will do the workouts, and you can also post them on your daily planner. It's a way of making an appointment with yourself and scheduling *you* into your day. There is something about writing down a goal and a time to accomplish it that makes it official.

Ideally, make your exercise appointment early in the day. I've found with my clients that as the day goes on, their resolve to work out becomes a fading dream and probably just won't happen. Morning is better, because my own research shows that you will exercise more frequently with better consistency and won't blow it off. If you're not a "morning person," go to bed half an hour earlier each night. I promise that you will feel great by starting your day with exercise and knowing that you "got it over with" and now can move on to other tasks.

If you let your exercise go until after dinner, chances are you won't do it. I've found it's iffy at best. You won't want to do it because it's late or cold or the laundry is waiting or you just sat down on the couch for five minutes, which turned into two hours and a quick nap. Or your favorite TV show is on, or you need to do homework with the kids . . . and then it's bath time. If you wait until 9 P.M. when everyone else is sleeping, your exercise routine will actually derail your program, because it will leave you too revved up to sleep. In a later chapter, I will explain how sleep is crucial for your success. (Yes, you're welcome on that one!)

The exercise sessions are short, and I promise that your spirits will soar if you do them when the day is new and full of promise.

Feel motivated? Got your picture? Got your workout area set up? Shoes laced up? Spirits revved up? Okay, good. Now it's time to fix your eating habits.

2. Feed 'Em—Part 1

It's time for a food wake-up call. What, how, and when you eat tells your body if it should store or burn fat for fuel and if it should build muscle or waste it.

The human body is the ultimate chemistry lab. What fools most people who fail on weight loss plans is believing in this non-fact: it's calories in, calories out. Think about it this way: if your body were simply a bank account, you could just divide up Snickers bars all day and have a "balanced" sugar party. You could eat doughnuts as your three meals and have great delts! Good luck with that!

My plan will turn you into a fat-burning machine. To accomplish this, you must follow my Virgin Rules of Meal Timing, which are:

- Eat a substantial breakfast within an hour of waking up.
- Stop eating three hours before bed (and no, this doesn't mean going to bed later!)
- Eat every four to six hours, which means you will be eating three balanced meals per day and at most one snack—and only if necessary. Promise me right now to stop all of that silly snacking.

If you are clutching those 100-calorie snack packs, I want you to consider this fact: every time you down one of those 100-calorie carb bombs, you raise your blood sugar level and subsequently your insulin level. When your insulin level is raised, the message to your body is to lock the doors to your fat cells and stop burning fat, as you have enough sugar in your blood stream to fuel your body. If you're eating every two to three hours, your body doesn't need to burn stored fat for fuel. Your goal is to burn that stored fat.

My program is not about deprivation. I promise that you will be so completely satisfied eating your meals that you won't even crave a snack. Please know that I'm not about to switch you off everything you love and put you on the tree-bark-and-lettuce plan. You will eat delicious, real foods that will be easy to prepare or to order if you like to eat out.

I focus on two concepts that will ensure your success without leaving you cranky and craving. The first thing is "add before you take away" by putting in more nonstarchy veggies, upping your fiber intake, and drinking water in between meals. The second is to make what I call "lateral shifts" with your daily faves so you won't instantly miss the foods you eat now. Then we'll work on trading up, so you can eat the healthiest diet possible that delivers maximum energy.

armed and dangerous

Stop listening to your girlfriends and your favorite celebrities for your eating plan. The ability to chew doesn't make someone a junior nutritionist. Your friend Vickie is not a nutritionist. And neither is Jessica Alba.

JJ's Perfect Eating Plate

From now on, you're going to eat according to my plate. It's an easy way to stay on this plan. It focuses on lean protein, healthful fats, nonstarchy veggies, and high-fiber, low-glycemic-index carbs. Why these? Because all four are essential to your health. Before you pick up a fork, remember that even with healthy foods, too much of a good thing turns it into a bad thing! If you consume too many calories, they have to go somewhere, and unfortunately that usually means into those pesky fat cells in your gut, butt, thighs, or arms. We want to get rid of your fat in order to lean out your body and sculpt your arms. My perfect eating plate will help you visualize portion control.

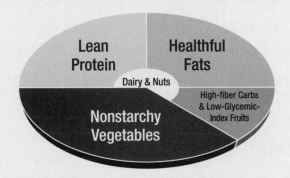

Picture a dinner plate divided into four sections. The top half will be equally divided between lean protein and healthy fats. The bottom half will be made up of three-quarters non-starchy vegetables and one-fourth high-fiber carbs and low-glycemic-index fruits. We'll be examining each food category in detail throughout the chapter.

My Eating Plan

This is one of the easiest eating plans in the world because you will eat within an hour of waking up, you will eat three meals a day every four to six hours, and you will stop eating three hours before bed. There will be one optional snack if you have to go for a longer period between your meals. You will eat breakfast, lunch, and dinner, with this one caveat: *You don't have to eat breakfast foods for breakfast.*

You will also eat what I call healthy and clean meals. This means every meal will include a lean protein, one serving of a high-fiber carb, *loads* of nonstarchy veggies, and some healthful fat. I'll explain them in detail in just a minute.

Here's a quick overview: protein is what we need to help us build muscle and will be eaten at every single meal because it's critical to your success. It slows down stomach emptying, which means that it keeps the hunger-triggering hormone ghrelin, which is produced by your stomach when it is empty, at bay. The right types of fat are some of the most therapeutic things you can add to your plate, as they support good brain function and mood, help with bone remodeling, and can reduce inflammation. When fat enters your small intestine, it also triggers the release of cholecystokinin (CCK), which tells your body that you are full, thus flipping off your appetite switch.

Finally, the right high-fiber carbs and nonstarchy veggies give your brain the energy you need to make it through the day. The fiber in these two groups also helps slow down stomach emptying, keeping you feeling fuller longer. As an added bonus, the fiber will give you poops you can be proud of. Yes, I just said that in my book because it's important that your body function in all the right (and regular—pun intended) ways. Plus, when you eat from the rainbow of fruits and veggies, you will get a plethora of great phytonutrients (plant nutrients) that can benefit you in a variety of ways, including giving you more energy, clearer skin, and less pain and inflammation. If you're on one of those stressful no-carb diets, a new day is about to dawn for you and you will love the sudden zap in your daily mojo because those no-carb plans leave people cranky, tired, and listless.

Again, the concept is that food provides information to your body. It dictates whether you store fat and burn sugar or burn fat and build muscle. You don't want to be a sugar burner, because then you won't reach your goals when it comes to your arms or any other part of your body.

By the way, I won't be asking you to whip up gourmet meals because, frankly, who has the time? And most of us aren't ready to go all Martha Stewart on a daily basis. These meals are simple, fast choices that do the trick.

A few general guidelines when choosing your meals:

- Eat 4 to 6 ounces of protein at each meal. That's approximately .75 to 1 gram per pound of fat-free mass. You can approximate this with the following formula:

    - Men, multiply your weight in pounds by 0.8 (0.85 if you are fit).

- Women, multiply your weight in pounds by 0.7 (0.8 if you are fit).

This will give you the total number of grams you should eat in a day. Divide this number by three to get the amount in each meal.

- Eat two or more servings of nonstarchy vegetables at each meal—the more, the better. A serving is 1 cup raw or ½ cup cooked; increase the number of servings to increase weight loss. Note that the *minimum* number of servings per day of these is five; your goal is ten!

- Eat one to three servings of fat at each meal. A serving is approximately 1 tablespoon of nut butter or oil, 10 small nuts, ⅓ of an avocado, ¼ cup of light coconut milk, 3 to 4 ounces of fish. Stick with two servings for accelerated fat loss.

- Eat one to two servings of high-fiber starchy carbs or fruits at each meal. A serving is 1 slice of bread, ½ cup of cooked grains, ⅓ cup of beans, ½ medium yam or sweet potato, ½ cup of winter squash, 1 apple, 1 cup of berries, or a sliced tomato. Stick with one serving per meal for accelerated fat loss, and if you want to skip your dinner serving, increase your intake of nonstarchy vegetables by at least two additional servings. Make sure to have at least one serving at breakfast and lunch so your brain is well fueled throughout the day!

- Don't forget to drink 8 to 12 glasses of water a day between meals. Drink only 4 to 8 ounces of water with meals because you don't want to dilute your stomach acid and impair your digestion.

Protein

Protein is crucial to a solid eating plan and necessary for losing weight and sculpting your arms. A little science first: protein slows down stomach emptying, which causes ghrelin to be suppressed so that you feel fuller longer. It also helps balance your insulin response when you eat carbohydrates. Studies indicate that when you replace some of your carbs with protein, you will naturally lose weight because your appetite will decrease—and rather quickly.

The rule is to consume .75 to 1 gram of protein per pound of fat-free mass per day. (This is why it's important to determine your ideal body mass as soon as possible.) Most women need about 4 to 6 ounces of protein at each meal. Your goal is to eat the highest-quality protein from animal sources. Remember, you are what you eat, so be sure to choose organic meats from animals such as grass-fed beef and wild fish that are fed what is natural to them.

What are good protein choices? Here are a few suggestions:

- Chicken and turkey breast (look for organic, free-range fowl)
- Grass-fed beef (go for lean cuts such as filet)

- Organic, cage-free eggs

- Organic, low-fat (not *non*fat) cottage cheese or ricotta cheese

- Feta or goat cheese

- Game

- Lamb

- Whey protein (cool-processed, and from grass-fed cows)

- Greek-style yogurt, because it has a higher protein content than regular yogurt

Protein Cheat Sheet

Knowing that you need to eat around 4–6 ounces of protein at each meal, here is a quick way to determine an average serving.

- Red meat: 7–9 grams of protein per ounce

- Turkey white meat: 9.5 grams per ounce

- Chicken white meat: 9.5 grams per ounce

- Fish: 7–9 grams per ounce

- Shellfish: 6–7 grams per ounce

- Whole eggs: 6.2 grams per ounce

- Feta cheese: 4 grams per ounce

- Cottage cheese: 15 grams per ounce (½ cup)

- Greek-style plain yogurt: 15–18 grams per 8 ounces

- Cold-water fish and shellfish. Look for wild fish. Ideal choices are salmon, sardines, scallops, sole, and halibut. Avoid farm-raised fish, which are subjected to herbicides, fungicides, and hormones and are fed a nonnative diet that changes their natural omega-3 fatty acids.
- Pea, rice, and hemp protein blends

Carbs

You shouldn't be carb-phobic anymore, but you do need to be conscious of the *best carbs* for your success. The best high-fiber carbs *aren't* white (bread, potatoes, rice, cakes, and all their cousins, such as cereal bars). The key is to have a high-fiber, low-glycemic-index carb with slower sugar release that keeps a steady supply of energy going to your brain.

The foundation of the U.S. Food Guide Pyramid is carbs, which is strange considering that though we can't live without protein, fat, or water, we can live without carbs (though we might get a bit cranky). You feel better when you eat carbs to keep a steady supply of blood sugar to your brain. The goal is to release the sugar slowly, which is what happens when you eat high-fiber carbs. This is the way to get that slow burn while keeping your blood sugar in check and avoiding insulin spikes. You will feel better for a longer time and will be able to go longer between meals. The end result of eating this way is using stored fat for fuel and losing weight.

Notice that I put nonstarchy veggies and low-glycemic-index fruits into a class all by themselves on your plate. While I am limiting your high-fiber, starchy carb intake, I want you to go full out on the nonstarchy veggies!

What are nonstarchy vegetables? They include:

- Arugula
- Beet greens
- Broccoli
- Cauliflower
- Lettuce (but not iceberg!)
- Snow peas
- Summer squashes
- Watercress
- Asparagus
- Brussels sprouts
- Celery
- Collard greens
- Eggplant
- Jalapeño peppers
- Mushrooms
- Radishes
- Shallots
- Swiss chard
- Bell peppers (red, yellow and green)

- Cabbages
- Endive
- Green beans
- Kale
- Mustard greens
- Radicchio
- Spinach
- Bean sprouts
- Cucumbers
- Fennel
- Kohlrabi
- Onions
- Spaghetti squash
- Turnip greens

Here are my favorite high-fiber, starchy carb choices:

- Jicama
- Squashes (acorn, butternut, and other winter squashes)
- Lima beans (okay, I hate them, but you might like 'em)
- Turnips
- Black beans
- Great Northern beans
- Navy beans
- Yellow beans

- Bulgur wheat (aka tabouli)
- Steel-cut oats
- Whole grains
- Whole-grain tortillas
- Lentils
- Legumes: chickpeas, kidney beans, split peas, white beans, etc.
- Barley
- Millet
- Ak-mak crackers
- Artichokes
- Pumpkin
- Brown rice
- Rye
- Whole-grain breads
- Ezekiel bread
- Yams
- Sweet potatoes
- Buckwheat (kasha)
- Whole-grain cooked cereals
- Wasa crackers

Most of my clients see the best results from living gluten-free, which means eliminating foods containing grains from their diet completely. Gluten can hurt your gastrointestinal tract and make it leaky, which impairs digestion and triggers other food sensitivities. Try the following gluten-free grains: rice, millet, amaranth, quinoa, teff, corn (must be non-GMO/organic), and buckwheat (kasha). Oatmeal is also gluten-free but is often grown near or processed in plants where gluten-containing grains are, so if you are very gluten-sensitive, be sure to look for a brand with "gluten free" on the label.

Fruits

Fruits fall under the high-fiber, starchy carb category. I highly recommend berries, as they are the lowest-glycemic-index fruits, loaded with fiber and antioxidants, and the perfect addition to your daily shake. Limit yourself to two fruit servings per day from the low- and moderate-glycemic-index lists. Remember to count these into your high-fiber, starchy carb servings. Think of the high-glycemic-index fruits as a treat, as in *dessert*!

Lowest-Glycemic-Index Fruits

- Berries

Moderate-Glycemic-Index Fruits

- Apples
- Cherries
- Grapefruit

- Pears
- Peaches
- Apricots
- Nectarines
- Kiwifruit
- Passion fruit
- Lemons
- Limes
- Persimmons
- Avocados
- Nectarines
- Plums
- Melons (except for watermelon)
- Oranges

armed and dangerous

Skip the juice. You wouldn't sit down and consume four to six oranges at a clip, but you can easily do so with a glass of juice! Plus you miss the fiber, the best part of the fruit, when you guzzle the juice.

High-Glycemic-Index Fruits

- Bananas
- Mangos
- Pineapple

- Papaya
- Grapes
- Watermelon
- Dried fruits
- Figs

Eat from the Rainbow

A great way to get maximum nutrients from your nonstarchy carbs is to eat from the rainbow. Some of the highest-nutrient-level and brightest-colored foods include:

- *Orange:* carrots, sweet potato, cantaloupe
- *Green:* broccoli, spinach, avocado
- *Red:* beets, red peppers, raspberries, pomegranate, cranberries, cherries
- *Blue:* blueberries
- *Purple:* red onion, radicchio
- *Black:* blackberries, olives, seaweed

Remember, always choose the organic varieties.

armed and dangerous

With self-awareness, you can apply my eating plan almost any-where. There are even healthful fast-food choices. If you visit Chipotle Grill, for instance, you can order a salad with black beans, chicken, guacamole, salsa, peppers, and onions. Use the salsa as your dressing. You just hit a healthy home run!

- High-fiber carbs: salsa, beans
- Nonstarchy veggies: peppers, onions, romaine
- Clean, lean protein: chicken
- Healthy fat: guacamole

Healthful Fats: Make an Oil Change

It's time to get over the fear of fat because fat doesn't make you fat. In fact, you *need* fat in your diet to burn your stored fat. Any healthful fat will help you attain great arms because it triggers the release of CCK, a neuropeptide that tells your brain that you are full, when it hits the small intestine. You also need it to build your bones and create gorgeous, strong, young-looking skin, hair, and nails. By the way, your brain is more than 50 percent fat. If you want to enjoy solid and clear thinking, you need fat. It may also help you avoid depression.

All fats are not created equal. Be careful not to eat trans fats or partially hydrogenated oils. Trade your corn oil for extra-virgin olive oil. And check the dates on your fat products because you certainly don't want to eat oils that have become rancid because they sat on the supermarket shelf or in your pantry for too long.

You want to choose monounsaturated fats and omega-3 polyunsaturated fats and coconut oil. A few suggestions:

- Extra-virgin olive oil
- Avocados
- Raw nuts and seeds
- Coconut milk/oil/meat
- Wild cold-water fish

Note: Peanuts are not nuts, so put down the can right now. They are legumes, so make an oil change from peanut butter to almond, cashew, or walnut butter—delish!

How to Make Lateral Shifts

I don't believe in diets because they are generally about deprivation. I prefer to have you make lateral shifts. You're not going to deny yourself the foods you love from day 1 of this plan. Instead you will simply make shifts that are healthy but don't make you feel as if you're denying yourself what you really want on your plate or in your glass.

For example, if you're a soda junkie, it's easy to make a lateral shift to sparkling water with a twist, including lemon, lime, or, one of my favorites, a flavored Emergen-C vitamin packet (I love raspberry!).

Try these other healthy shifts:

- Trade sugar-loaded coffee drinks for plain coffee with a splash of coconut milk.
- Trade vegetable oil (safflower, sunflower, soybean, and corn oil) for extra-virgin olive oil, walnut oil, or sesame oil.
- Trade ready-made salad dressing for your own blend of extra-virgin olive oil and a specialty vinegar.
- Trade orange juice for a fresh orange.
- Trade sweetened iced black tea for iced green tea with fruit essence.
- Trade artificial sweetener and sugar for xylitol.
- Trade iceberg lettuce for spinach greens.
- Trade peanuts for almonds, walnuts, and pecans.
- Trade nutrient-depleted table salt for sea salt.
- Trade Egg Beaters for cage-free, organic eggs.
- Trade high-sugar fruit yogurts for plain Greek-style yogurt with berries, vanilla, or cinnamon.
- Trade white potatoes for yams or sweet potatoes.
- Trade mashed potatoes for mashed cauliflower.
- Trade blue cheese crumbles for goat cheese.

- Trade 80 percent lean hamburger for grass-fed beef patties or turkey or chicken breast patties.
- Trade corn-fed rib-eye steak for grass-fed filet mignon.
- Trade chicken thighs and wings for organic chicken breasts.
- Trade white rice for brown and wild rices, steamed in chicken broth.
- Trade farm-raised fish for wild fish.
- Trade sugar-loaded marinara sauce for organic, no-sugar-added marinara sauce.
- Trade light mayonnaise for gourmet mustard blends.
- Trade refried beans for fat-free pinto beans with Mexican seasoning.
- Trade fried taco shells for soft, whole-grain tortillas.
- Trade dried raisins for frozen grapes.
- Trade peanut butter for almond, cashew, macadamia, or walnut butter.
- Trade white pasta for whole wheat, quinoa, or rice pasta.
- Trade margarine for organic butter.
- Trade ketchup for salsa.
- Trade ranch dip for hummus.

Keep the Enemy out of the House

It follows that you don't want temptation staring you in the face. I love the study that indicated that people who kept a bowl of Hershey kisses on their desk ate nine per day; people a couple of

10 So-Called Healthy Foods You're Eating Now That Keep Your Arms Fat

- Diet cookies—they are still cookies.
- "Light" yogurt. It contains less fat but is still loaded with carbs and sugars.
- Frozen yogurt. It's making a comeback, but the yogurt part is BS. It's adult ice cream.
- Artificial nondairy coffee creamer. Chemicals in your coffee are not good!
- Sugar-free anything. Put that sugar-free pudding down right now.
- Microwave popcorn. It's full of damaged fats and toxic chemicals, *and* the corn is high-glycemic-index—a triple threat to your arms!
- Baked chips. Try no chips.
- 100-calorie snack packs. You're setting your body up to burn just sugar and not fat.
- "Healthy" muffin tops or bran muffins. Why not just eat cake? A muffin plus a latte averages 600 calories and is mainly sugar and carbs!
- Smoothies. Most people supersize them. Just say no.
- Flavored waters. Added sugar or artificial sweeteners make a good thing bad!

- Artificial sweeteners. Research shows that these cause "calorie dysregulation," which in plain English means they may cause you to overeat!
- "Diet" bars and so-called energy bars. They're essentially adult candy bars.

desks away ate only three. It's very clear that we respond to food triggers. Why do you think Starbucks has that pastry case in your face the moment you walk in the store? It wants you to be overcome by those banana nut muffins.

Don't rely on willpower and make things hard for yourself. Remember that late at night your evil twin will come out and remind you where the chocolate chip cookies are hiding. If sweets are in the big smelly trash can outside, you won't eat them. And please stop with the excuse that you need to keep bad things in the house for your kids. When you don't buy doughnuts for the household, you're actually doing all of you a major favor and giving everyone's health a big boost. If you must bring a few enemies into the house, at least get the snacks that *you* don't really enjoy. If your husband needs his stash, suggest that he keep it in a locked box. Every little bit helps nudge you toward success. (By the way, if he needs chips or he will stop breathing and you hate Doritos but love Cheetos, by all means buy him the former. The best idea, however, would be for both of you to skip the chips. Sorry, but I had to say it!)

In the next chapter I will teach you how to retrain your taste buds for good so that you won't even want the items that we just threw into the trash. I will also focus on some meal plans that are simple, tasty, and filling.

3. Feed 'Em—Part 2 (Meal Plans)

So you're making the lateral eating shifts and your plate has changed from a carb-bomb mess to lean protein, nonstarchy vegetables, a high-fiber carb, and some healthy fat. You start to wonder if you were kidnapped by aliens and mind-melded because you're actually craving spinach. It seems strange at first, but you can't wait to get those berries into a bowl.

Congrats, because you're retraining your taste buds!

Eventually you will be able to be at a party, eat a few bites of cake, and not wreck your program because the cake won't even taste that great. Why? Again, you have done a major "makeover" of your taste buds. I know someone who was a Diet Coke-a-holic and went off the stuff for three months. By accident, she grabbed someone else's glass, thought the Diet Coke was iced tea, and was revolted by the taste. This is a woman who used to down a six-pack a day and told me she couldn't live without the stuff.

Believe me when I say that it's groundbreaking and personally freeing to retrain your taste buds to not even like the foods that you were addicted to just a few months ago. You will move away from your addiction to sweet and shift to a love of savory and spicy. It's much better to love salsa as a dip than creamy ranch dressing or sugary sweet-and-sour sauce. One day it will dawn on you that sugary and creamy aren't even your choice sensations anymore. You really do want the spicy.

Perhaps you've retasted some of those weird-tasting, chemical-crappy foods packed with artificial sweeteners that now taste so fake and bitter. You grabbed a so-called health bar or a diet cookie and were revolted because it tasted phony and plastic. This is the ultimate freedom and the way you will stay on this plan forever. It's as if you finally flipped a switch, which will make your plan an unstoppable one.

Meal Planning

It helps to spell things out a bit when you start a new plan, so I'm offering some specific meal plans that you can follow or mix and match according to the plate in the previous chapter. The following ideas will help you plan each meal in a simple, effective way. Soon this will be second nature to you.

Breakfast

Forget about skipping breakfast. Numerous studies show that eating a substantial breakfast with optimal protein is essential for fat loss and long-term weight management. This equates to approximately 400 to 600 calories. Breakfast sets your metabolic tone for the day, which will dictate how well you are able to sustain your energy and burn fat for fuel. Don't fall into the old breakfast trap and have just a muffin or yogurt. You need optimal protein to prevent a midmorning blood sugar crash. The traditional cereal and milk is a carb bomb that sets you up to detonate around 10 A.M.

Here are a few great breakfast choices:

- Nutty oatmeal with long-cooking steel-cut oats. Add cinnamon, vanilla, 1–2 tablespoons chopped nuts, and 1–2 scoops vanilla whey protein. You can also have two poached eggs on the side for the protein instead of the whey.
- Cottage cheese with 1 cup of strawberries and 2 tablespoons chopped almonds.
- No-hormones added turkey slices (4–6 ounces) from the deli, a corn tortilla, and ½ avocado. Make into a wrap and add leftover grilled veggies from last night.

- Breakfast out: three-egg veggie omelet with sliced ⅓ avocado and a cup of fresh berries.

One of my favorite ways to tackle breakfast is with a shake. It's simple, easy, and packed with everything you need, plus delicious. Read on!

How to Create the Perfect Shake

Studies show that when you replace one meal a day with a healthy balanced shake you will lose more weight and keep it off. I'm a big fan of shakes because you can shove nutrition into them and they're easy to make, drink, and even take on the road with you. Of course, I'm not talking about putting some frozen vanilla yogurt with artificial sweeteners, juice, and a banana into the blender. That's not a healthy shake, and neither are the shakes you buy from most places even when they claim that they're healthful. It's best if you make the shake and follow a few simple rules:

- You won't put any artificial sweeteners in the shake. I prefer xylitol or stevia. If you use fructose, it must be 5 grams or less per serving. Don't be fooled by "all-natural" sweeteners, as they are still all sugar and some, such as agave, are high in fructose. You should avoid them.

- Depending on how much protein you need for the day, I'd suggest between 25 and 40 grams. Most women need about 25 to 30 grams total (you will get a little from any added nuts or flax as well). Protein sources include cool-processed whey, pea, rice, or hemp. Avoid soy protein and straight milk or egg powders.

    Note: Not all whey is created equal! Look for cool-processed whey—ideally from cows fed grass and not shot up with hormones, antibiotics, and the like! Don't go looking for the best bargain tub at the wholesale club. See Resources for the ones I use and recommend to my clients.

Shake Steps

1. Pick a protein.
2. Add fiber.
3. Add a healthful fat.
4. Add fruit.
5. Add water and ice to create the desired thickness.

armed and dangerous

I've been a big fan of shakes for fifteen years now. I do them for breakfast and sometimes even do two shakes a day, depending on what's going on. Six days out of seven, I have a shake for one meal a day. When I'm traveling, I take my Magic Bullet blender and skip the $50 room service charge for eggs. It irritates me to spend so much for what's basically a $6 breakfast. I even carry shaker cups onto a plane if I will need a meal while flying. Just put the shake mix into the cup and then ask for water once you're in your seat. It's an easy way to stay on the plan.

My Favorite Shake Recipe

- 1–2 scoops protein powder.
- 1–2 servings of fiber (see Resources for my favorite fiber blend, Essential Fiber by Metabolic Maintenance; other great choices are Salba Rx and freshly ground flaxseed meal). A serving should give you 5 or more grams of fiber. Flax and Salba also contain healthful fat.
- 1–2 servings of healthful fat, such as 1 tablespoon organic nut butter (not peanut) or ¼ cup light coconut milk (replaces ¼ cup of water).
- 1 cup frozen organic berries.
- 1 cup pure spring water.

Blend. Add ice and blend again to achieve the desired thickness.

armed and dangerous

Coconut milk helps you lose fat! It can aid fat burning, lower your appetite, and boost your metabolism. Plus it tastes great!

Lunch and Dinner

Now that you're into the groove of the plan, it's easy to figure out the lunch and dinner choices, which really are endless. Just put together your clean, lean proteins, healthful fats, nonstarchy veggies, and a high-fiber, starchy carb. A salad of greens and veggies with an olive oil vinaigrette for healthful fat is always a great starter. Plus the vinegar helps slow down the blood sugar response and makes your insulin receptors more sensitive, which means better fat burning and more sustained energy.

One of my lunch favorites is a wrap sandwich. It's easy to eat at work and won't get soggy by noon. Really load up your wrap

How to Wrap It Right

1. Choose a protein.

2. Add nonstarchy veggies.

3. Add a healthful fat, such as avocado, olive oil, raw nuts, or seeds.

4. Roll it all up in a whole-grain wrap.

Remember never to wrap in a white-flour tortilla. Choose a whole-grain tortilla or a whole wheat pita. Add a side salad or some carrot and celery sticks. You don't need fruit because you already have your carb—the actual wrap.

with a rainbow of nonstarchy veggies, including spinach, cucumbers, peppers, red onions, and so on. Add last night's leftover protein, and throw in some avocado for a healthful fat. Or you can add nuts and seeds to the wrap to give it a little more crunch.

armed and dangerous

Need a quick lunch or dinner that you can freeze for later portions? Make a great veggie and protein soup. Start with an organic chicken or veggie broth and add your favorite cooked protein. Throw in nonstarchy veggies and legumes. Cover and cook over medium heat until veggies and legumes are cooked through, 25 to 30 minutes. This soup gets better the next day as the flavors "marry." Serve it with a salad with olive oil vinaigrette and some chopped nuts or avocado, and you have a fast, inexpensive, hearty lunch that's a complete meal. Best of all, you'll have extra servings to freeze that will save you when you're too busy to cook.

Veggies and Salads

Jazz up your veggies to keep them interesting. Try roasting them, sautéing them, or sprinkling chopped nuts over them. I love to add Mexican, Asian, or Italian seasonings to veggies. Roasting them in a little bit of extra-virgin olive oil is always tasty, and I make more than I need for future wraps and meals. Extra roasted veggies are also great in a salad. Preheat the oven to 400 degrees. Just line them up on a cookie sheet, drizzle with extra-virgin olive oil, add a little ground black pepper and sea salt, and toss. You can also sprinkle on herbs such as rosemary and garlic for extra flavor. Check veggies at 20 minutes, turn them over, and roast for another 20 or more minutes. Cooking time will vary depending on size of vegetable pieces. Roast red peppers and onions in the veggie mix because they're especially yummy and loaded with phytonutrients.

As for salads, you want to ditch the store-bought dressings even if they profess to be healthy. Just buy delicious vinegar and a great olive oil. Add herbs such as rosemary or basil and mix in a bit of Dijon mustard. Use one to two parts oil to one part vinegar. It's easy to make your own dressing, and you can even use a bit as a healthful fat in your wraps.

It's important to create the most healthful salad possible that's also delicious. Here are a few ways I like to build a great salad.

Create the Foundation

Start with 2 or more cups of the following (the more the better!): romaine, cabbage, mixed greens, baby greens, radicchio, endive, or watercress. Add some nonstarchy veggies such as asparagus, onions, peppers, radishes, cucumbers, mushrooms, and leftover roasted veggies.

Pile on Some Protein

Add 4 to 6 ounces of protein depending on your weight and activity level and the amount of fat in the item. The higher the fat content, the more the ounces, and count it as a healthful fat serving as well. Pick your protein: grilled chicken, sliced turkey breast, grass-fed beef, wild salmon, halibut, scallops, shrimp, or hard-boiled eggs.

Fuel It with Fats

Add some healthful fats: olives, nuts (not candied or glazed), goat cheese, avocado, organic extra-virgin olive oil, sesame oil, walnut oil, grapeseed oil, or wild fish.

Fill Up with Fiber

Add some high-fiber carbs: lentils, black beans, garbanzo beans, jicama, sweet potato, brown rice, tomato, brown rice cakes, RyKrisp (on the side or crumbled in), apple chunks, mandarin oranges (*not* in syrup), berries, or grapefruit segments.

Spice It Up

Spice it up with a yummy-flavored vinegar (check to make sure it doesn't contain sugar), fresh herbs (I love fresh basil), gourmet mustard, sea salt, freshly ground pepper, light soy sauce, sliced gingerroot, or red pepper flakes.

My Quick Salad Dressing

1 tablespoon olive, walnut, sesame, or grapeseed oil

1 tablespoon rice wine, pomegranate, red wine,
champagne, or balsamic vinegar

Spice it up with red onion, fresh garlic, herbes de Provence, Italian
herb mix, fresh basil, fresh thyme, lemon juice, gourmet mustard,
sea salt, cracked black pepper. Get creative.

My Favorite Salad Recipes

Mexican Tostada-less Salad

2 cups chopped romaine lettuce

1 cup total thinly sliced peppers, onions, and radishes

6 ounces grilled chicken

1 tablespoon salsa

⅓ cup cooked black beans

1 tablespoon guacamole

Combine the ingredients in a salad bowl.

Dressing

1 tablespoon olive oil

1 tablespoon red wine vinegar

Mix together and toss with a salad in a bowl.

Asian Salad

6 ounces grilled scallops

2 cups total butter lettuce and green cabbage mix

1 cup total julienned carrots, julienned red pepper, radish slices

¼ cup mandarin oranges

1 brown rice cake crumbled over the top

1 tablespoon sliced almonds

Combine the ingredients in a salad bowl.

Dressing

1 tablespoon sesame oil

1 tablespoon rice wine vinegar

1 teaspoon sesame seeds

1 teaspoon grated orange rind

1 shake red pepper flakes

Blend ingredients together and toss with the salad.

Summer Salad

2-plus cups total butter leaf lettuce and radicchio

1 cup total chopped cucumbers, sliced red onions,
and blanched and chilled asparagus cut into 1-inch segments

½ cup pink grapefruit segments

6 ounces cooked jumbo shrimp

⅓ avocado, sliced

Combine the ingredients in a salad bowl.

Dressing

1 tablespoon walnut oil

1 tablespoon rice wine vinegar

Blend together and toss with the salad.

Spinach Salad

2 or more cups fresh spinach leaves

1 cup sliced cucumber, mushrooms, and red onions

1 tablespoon chopped pecans

1 tablespoon goat cheese crumbles

½ cup strawberries

½ cup julienned jicama

4–6 ounces grass-fed beefsteak, grilled rare and sliced

Combine the ingredients in a salad bowl.

Dressing

1 tablespoon olive oil

1 tablespoon pomegranate vinegar

Blend together and toss with the salad.

Winter Salad

2-plus cups mixed greens

¼ cup torn basil leaves

1 cup roasted veggies

½ cup cooked garbanzo beans

1 tablespoon chopped walnuts

Combine the ingredients in a salad bowl.

Dressing

1 tablespoon olive oil

1 tablespoon balsamic vinegar

1 teaspoon gourmet ground mustard

Blend together and toss with the salad. Top with 6 ounces warmed grilled salmon.

Wrap It Up

1 whole-grain wrap or whole-grain pita

1 cup mixed greens and veggies

4–6 ounces protein

Choose one: ⅓–½ avocado, 2 tablespoons raw nuts or seeds,
or 2 ounces goat cheese

Spice it up. Ideally, serve with crudités or a side salad, as you can fit
only so many veggies into a wrap!

Additional Ideas for a Perfect Lunch or Dinner

We've already tossed some amazing salads that make great lunches and dinners. I'd like to offer you several other meals that you can make easily. One of my favorites is a large pot of soup. It's so easy to take to the office in a thermos and is a great fast meal at night.

Souper Meal

Organic veggie or chicken broth

Your favorite nonstarchy veggies, such as zucchini,
onions, peppers, mushrooms, and so on

Add a high-fiber carb, such as a root veggie, legumes, or brown and wild rice. It should provide a ½-cup serving per 2-to-3-cup serving of soup/stew.

Pick a protein—you can mix it up here.

Combine all the ingredients in a Crock-Pot. Cook for 2 hours on high heat or for 6–8 hours on low heat. If you don't have a Crock-Pot, combine all the ingredients in a stockpot, bring to a boil over high heat, cover, lower the heat, then simmer for 25–30 minutes or until the veggies are fork tender and your protein is cooked through.

Serve with a salad with olive oil vinaigrette or crudités with guacamole.

Foundational Meal

Start with a salad with extra-virgin olive oil and vinegar.

Pick a protein.

Add nonstarchy veggies.

Fill up with a high-fiber carb.

Fuel with healthful fats.

Sample Menus

Mixed green salad with extra-virgin olive oil vinaigrette

Grilled halibut on a bed of spinach and
mushrooms sautéed in olive oil

½ cup mixed brown and wild rice, chicken broth

....

Romaine salad with cucumbers, celery, radishes,
and extra-virgin olive oil vinaigrette

Grilled chicken

Roasted veggies

Sweet potato with cinnamon and chopped
pecans roasted at 350° for an hour

....

Gazpacho topped with fresh sliced avocado

Grilled grass-fed beefsteak topped with
sautéed mushrooms and onions

Asparagus and red pepper medley sautéed in olive oil

Optional Snack and Emergency Foods

I always have emergency food on me so I don't get stuck. Just
grab a baggie and take along 10 to 20 nuts, an apple, and a shake

mix that's already in the shaker cup and just needs water added. Avoid those fake "health" bars. Most are candy bars in disguise, and they're terrible for you. I have checked them all out, and there is only *one* that I use myself and let my clients have: Paleo-bars (see Resources for the lowdown). Make sure you always tote your emergency food, and you will never face having to make the best choice from the worst offerings.

What, No Dessert?

Berries are your best dessert choice. If you have a sweet tooth, 1 to 2 ounces of 80% or higher dark chocolate will do the trick. Please don't keep the chocolate in the house. I have already tested that theory for you, and I can promise you, you will eat the whole bar. Don't rely on your willpower; rely on your logic, and get the enemy out of the house! And though dark chocolate definitely has some health benefits due to its high antioxidant content, it also packs a wallop of calories, sugar, and fat in a teeny-weeny serving, so it's easy to go overboard. Make it special, so you appreciate it as a treat!

Don't worry about missing dessert, because as you retrain your taste buds you will lose the taste for it. All of a sudden, you will eat a bite of something sweet and it will be so sweet that you won't even like it because it makes your tongue curdle and your stomach hurt and you actually feel your blood sugar surge.

What Do I Eat after Dinner?

The answer is: nothing!

The rule is that you don't eat at all for three hours before you go to bed. Replace the needless snacking with sex, a bath, or a walk.

Most people eat late at night out of sheer boredom. If you're still hungry after dinner, you did something wrong and didn't eat enough that day. When you eat late at night and go to bed with a full stomach, you keep your ghrelin suppressed. This is the hormone that you want to keep suppressed during the day so you aren't hungry, but at night, while you are sleeping, it should be at its highest level, as it correlates with a good growth hormone response. Better growth hormone response means better fat burning, more muscle building, and putting the skids on cellular aging.

What Do I Drink?

Let's start with what you won't be drinking. I want you to ban *all* artificial sweeteners from your life, and this includes what you drink. In a calorie dysregulation study, rats were given sugar water and then rat food. They ate what they needed to maintain their weight. Then the same rats were given artificially sweetened water, and again they ate what they needed to maintain their weight. The problem arose when the rats went back to the sugar water, as they could no longer correlate the degree of sweetness with the amount of calories, so they overate.

When you eat sweet, you crave sweet. You're in the process of retraining your taste buds to perceive a blueberry or an apple as delicious and sweet. This will be impossible to do if you keep confusing your taste buds into thinking that artificially supersweetened jam is the level of sweetness that sets the bar. The same goes for that light cranberry juice with a name-brand artificial sweetener that's so sweet it tosses you into a sugar coma. Again, this sets a range of sweetness that throws your taste buds into a sugar-craving frenzy.

Add potential toxicity and an evil accelerated aging process called glycation to the list of potential bad things that artificial sweeteners do. To sum up, there is nothing I can say about artificial sweeteners that's healthy or positive.

If you must use one, my favorite sweetener is xylitol. It's an antibacterial sugar alcohol that's actually good for your bones and doesn't raise your blood sugar. It's also low on the glycemic index and slows stomach emptying, which can help with weight loss. If you eat too much of it, you will get gas and your body will force you to stop, which is another plus (I call it natural rate limiting.) A little bit of the naturally sweet herb stevia is fine too, but don't go crazy with it. Too much of it may cause the same calorie dysregulation phenomenon that I described with the rats.

Lateral Shift: Substitute Sparkling Water with Emergen-C for Soda

Just think of soda as poison and tell yourself you're not going to poison yourself anymore. Start by limiting yourself to one soda a day and replacing the others with water and sparkling water with an Emergen-C packet. I love to add the pink lemonade Emergen-C to sparkling water. Now you have a drink that's actually good for you! As you wean the soda out of your life, try a soda-free week. After a week of no soda, take a sip or two. Isn't it interesting that suddenly it tastes . . . really bad? You will get used to this soda-free life and stop craving it, and you will immediately appreciate the debloating effect of cutting out all that carbonation.

Don't go crazy with the sparkling water. Use it to wean yourself from your soda habit, and then enjoy it as your boost one to two times a day with your Emergen-C packet or as your "mocktail" when you are out. Too much carbonation makes you feel bloated, and that's never sexy.

For those of you who have lived on soda and didn't drink much water, this new way of drinking will really help you. You need water to burn fat. Diet soda is not water. You wouldn't put diet soda into the radiator of your car, and neither should you try to use diet soda in place of water in your body. It's very acidifying, and you actually need more water in your diet if you drink soda, to balance out the acid load. Still craving a soda? Try one just once a month. Soon enough you won't even want it anymore, I promise.

A Cup of Java

Hopefully, you will cut down on your coffee consumption, but you don't have to give it up. A small amount of coffee (organic, of course) is actually good for you. What you put into your coffee is what's key. I love a little bit of low-fat coconut milk, or you can add a tiny shot of organic cream or half-and-half. If you need a sweetener, use a bit of cinnamon, vanilla extract, or xylitol.

No Joy in Soy

Please, skip the soy milk in your coffee or as a drink (or in other foods). Along with corn, soy (unless it's organic) is one of the top genetically modified crops. You think you're choosing a healthy alternative, but you're not. It has been genetically modified to withstand spraying with pesticides. It is then processed in aluminum casks. Since soy contains fat, it is a great carrier of toxins. When you look at a lot of soy products, they are highly refined and contain loads of added sugar to boot. A high soy intake has been linked with lower thyroid function too. So if you are switching to soy products for health and weight loss, it could be backfiring on you.

Eating Out

The great news is that eating out is actually easier than eating in. First, you can't get up and go to the kitchen for seconds! And you really can control how you eat out with a few simple tips:

- Look at the menu as a guide and not an absolute. Let's say there's a great grilled salmon, but it comes with gooey risotto. But the chicken dish comes with a great Brussels sprouts side. (Yes, I really do like them.) You can easily mix and match what's on the menu. But first you must . . .
- Make waiters your friends and coconspirators. They will help you do what you want to do if you engage them. They can also tell you the great veggies that everyone loves and the best protein dish of the house and exactly how it's cooked.
- Remember, my plate guidelines don't change when you go out your front door.
- When I'm out, my rule is to have protein and a double order of veggies, plus some berries for dessert. It's a great way to obey the rules of the plate. Always start out with a colorful salad with olive oil and vinegar. But watch out for salad traps, including glazed nuts, dried fruit, croutons, and fattening blue cheese crumbles. Always

skip the creamy dressings. And remember that all vinaigrettes aren't created equal. Balsamic vinaigrette is fine, but a raspberry one is just packed with sugar, as are all those Asian dressings. Skip fried wontons in your salad too. Use common sense.

- Tell the waiter how to cook your protein (grilled, roasted, or baked), and ask which sauce it is served with. Keep all creamy sauces on the side, and avoid any fried meats. Barbecue sauce, plum sauce, and sweet-and-sour sauce are sugar nightmares. They're like putting sugar on your meat.

- Look for wild fish, grass-fed beef, or organic chicken.

- A great starter is the guacamole some restaurants make tableside, but ask the waiter to bring cut-up veggies with it so you can avoid the chips. Or try hummus with some cucumber slices. Just remember that starters count in your overall meal composition.

- Try veggies that you normally don't try at home. I had mustard greens recently at a restaurant, and they were delicious. Watch out for the prep and presentation when it comes to the veggies. You don't want to turn a great idea into a bad choice. Avoid anything called "crispy," which is usually a kinder way of saying fried. Make sure they aren't served in a creamy or sweet sauce. And obviously, tempura is a *no.*

- Don't turn your salad into a dessert. You must avoid salads with dried fruits and candied, sugared anything that just cranks up the calories. Don't throw 10 pounds of cheese on a salad. The starter salad shouldn't have more calories than the meal. You can add healthful fats such as plain nuts or avocado to your salad. For entrée salads, avoid fried chicken toppings, crispy noodles, and fried strips of anything, including tortilla strips. Remember that the vinegar in your dressing balances your blood sugar without loading you up with calories, so go for it. You can also put salsa and a little guacamole on your salad as dressing instead.

- Navigate a salad bar by choosing veggies, mixed greens, and legumes plus other proteins. Avoid anything in a sauce that's creamy, such as mayo. Add a few nuts, and use oil and vinegar.
- When you go out to eat, avoid the breadbasket at all costs.
- If you must eat something that's off the plan, use my three-bite rule.

JJ's Three Polite Bites Rule

If you say, "I'm never going to have X, Y, or Z again," of course you will crave it and think about it as if it's some past love that jilted you and now you're going to get it back. The three-bite rule will keep you on your game.

If you want a chocolate chip cookie and you try to replace it with some tasteless diet cookie, your craving will become worse. Once in a while—I repeat, *once in a while*, not every single day—you can have something you love, but only if you eat three ladylike bites of it.

Find what's really worth it to you. Maybe it is crusty bread or pizza, or the homemade tiramisù at your favorite Italian restaurant. Eat three polite bites as if you were being filmed while eating it for a national TV show. That means you're not shoveling it in.

After you've had your three bites, you're done. If you give yourself this permission, you will never pig out again and feel you have to eat every bite of a treat. But it is essential to allow yourself to eat the thing you really want and get over it. Share your treat with someone who has a fast fork. I take my three bites and then shove it out of arm's reach. A minute or two later, it's gone.

Alcohol and Your Arms

Of course, it's best if you skip alcoholic drinks, but you could also adopt my motto: Pinot Noir is your friend. I call it "the pretty drink." It's antiaging and anti-inflammatory. It's like taking your skin to the gym. Red wine is your best choice. The other two good options are tequila on the rocks with lime or a vodka martini (and have the olive—a great healthful fat). But this is *not Sex and the City,* so no Cosmos, gals. The cranberry cocktail juice (or similar sugar-loaded juice) that makes a Cosmo or other drinks pretty is truly treacherous. It's loaded with high-fructose corn syrup, the worst sugar you can consume.

Be careful overall with alcoholic beverages when you're out. Let's say someone orders a bottle of wine for the table. You might not even notice how often the waitress keeps refilling your glass and thus have no idea how much you drink. You also might have to deal with the peer pressure of a friend saying "Girl, you're not drinking. Let's relax and have fun!" You can easily say, "Oh, I have a presentation to give in the morning, so I'll just have a glass. But enjoy yourself."

As for other beverages, drink only 4 to 8 ounces of sparkling water or flat water with your meal. Too much water dilutes your stomach acid and you don't digest your food as well. You shouldn't be eating and drinking at the same time. Ideally, sit down and have a glass of sparkling water. By the time your food arrives in the form of a salad twenty minutes later, you're done drinking. Have a glass of wine with your meal and call it quits. If you want something else, go for an herbal tea with your dessert of fresh berries.

Now that we've been doing all of this good eating and drinking, it's time to move. I'm going to show you the best ways to work out, get strong, and sculpt your new arms.

4. Work 'Em

Are you ready to move? This is the chapter where we burn the fat and mold and sculpt your gorgeous new arms. Please don't blame me if the rest of your body suddenly starts taking on a new form and your jeans start falling off you. Get out the big bag for Goodwill, because soon your shirts will look like sacks and that great skirt you shimmied and tortured yourself to zip up last season will have the people in your life saying, "Did you lose weight? That skirt is hanging off you."

Enough talking. It's time to put on your shoes and sweats and hit the pavement, the gym, or that nice nook you've created in your house that is your private exercise zone.

By the way, in my program you spend much less time on

exercise than ever before because perhaps in the past you were walking an hour a session or lifting weights for what felt like for-ever.

With my program, you will get fit and your arms will get slim from spending the right *minutes* each week.

Let's go!

Burst to Burn Fat

Bursting is the key to your cardio workout on this program. This special type of training will get you fit in just minutes each week. It's the most effective and efficient way to teach your body to become a fat-burning machine. It's short but intense intervals of exercise done for just 30 to 60 seconds each. You won't get the limbs of your dreams just by lifting weights because you "hate cardio." I promise that you won't hate it anymore because my cardio bursting takes very little time and the intense portion is over with before you can blink. Think about it this way: don't you have four hard-core bursts in you? I know that most of you do.

Your mission with bursting is to work hard enough that you can't go a second longer. Think back to the relay races you did as a kid. You would line up on the playground and then run as hard as you could go to get to the finish line, tag your friend, and then you would have to rest for a minute or two. Your lungs were burn-ing, and your legs couldn't move one more millimeter.

As adults, we seldom have that exhilarating feeling. What makes you feel this way is lactic acid, a by-product created in your body when you use a lot of energy in a short time. When you raise your lactic acid levels, you trigger the release of human growth hormone (HGH). This is said to be "the hormone of youth" because it's at a high level when you are younger and helps you maintain muscle mass, burn fat, and keep your skin looking dewy and supple.

When you work at high intensity, you also use a lot of carbohydrates for fuel. Now, I know you're thinking: But wait, I want to burn body fat for fuel! Well, it turns out that when you burn more carbs during exercise, you store them back better after exercise (to give you energy for the next go-round tomorrow) and you burn more fat. After all, you are exercising for a short time each day, but you are living all day long; by exercising hard and burning more carbs during exercise, you teach your body how to burn more fat all day long, which has a much bigger impact on your metabolism and your body composition.

Because bursting is intense, it has a much bigger "metabolic cost" than walking or steady-state aerobic exercise. It creates an oxygen debt, which your body has to pay back after you are done exercising. What this means to your metabolism is that it has to work harder afterward to recover from the intense exercise you did. This doesn't happen after a daily walk. After all, that is just controlled falling, and your body is acclimated to walking about.

I want you to start by bursting in 30-to-60-second intervals to accumulate four total minutes every other day. You can increase to 8 minutes of total bursting as you increase your stamina. You will follow your burst by recovering for double that time—that is, 1 minute for every 30-second burst. I call this active recovery because you're still moving but you're not bursting. For example, you will sprint for 1 minute and then walk for 2 minutes. Or you will run up the stairs for 30 seconds and then walk down easy for a minute. Or jump rope hard for 1 minute and then walk around for 2 minutes. The easy recovery phase helps you buffer the lactic acid so you can go hard again in the next round. You will then be able to accumulate more lactic acid over the session, which will trigger a great growth hormone response. And the fitter you are, the longer that growth hormone stays around.

Don't use your heart rate as a guide, as by the time your heart rate gets high enough on the monitor, you should be long done! Instead, pay close attention to your exertion level.

Think of it this way: You work out on a scale of 1 to 10. When you burst, you should be in the 9–10 zone of toughness and exertion when you are finished. You should think you couldn't go another step. Some people might get to this point after 30 seconds, others after 45 or 60 seconds. That's fine as long as you're exerting yourself. If you feel you could burst for 90 seconds, you're not going hard enough. You should never be able to get past 60 seconds, and you should be slightly breathless. If you can talk on your cell phone while you are doing this, you're not bursting. You're not bursting on the bike at the gym if you can simultaneously work on a crossword puzzle.

To reiterate: you will never burst longer than 60 seconds. If you can get to 60 seconds and keep going, you need to increase your intensity. The adjustment might happen to you in a matter of days because your progress will be quite amazing and you will be blown away at how quickly you will be able to increase the intensity of your bursting.

As you continue to burst, you will find that other physically exerting challenges, such as running up and down the stairs in your house and racing after your kids, suddenly seem easy. Your energy throughout the day will soar too. Oh, and the scale will also start heading south because you'll be burning more fat than ever before.

Bursting Cheat Sheet

- Warm up for 3 minutes.
- Burst for 30–60 seconds.
- Recover for 1–2 minutes.
- Repeat to accumulate 4 total minutes of bursting (8 if you are already in great shape and want to take it to the next level).
- Cool down for 3 minutes.
- You're done. Really, you're done.

Great Ways to Burst

Below, I offer you some of my favorite bursting exercises. One is not better than the others, and it's always good to mix them up so your body doesn't adapt to any of them. Your goal is to keep progressing and improving by keeping your body guessing. One day I might do Turkish Get-ups (which honestly I hate, but I do them), and then the next session I'll do stair climbing. You can certainly do four 60-second bursts of anything you hate because the minutes will go by in a flash. Ideally, your aim isn't even to last the whole 60 seconds of the burst but to wipe yourself out as quickly as possible. You should be thinking, "Uggggh, enough" during the last 30 seconds—if you can make it.

I can't sprint because I have knee problems, so I remind you to please listen to your body's limitations. I like to do the StairMaster and the bike. Those of you who haven't exercised for a while may find a fast 60-second walk up a hill to be a burst. Figure out what's challenging for you!

My favorite bursting exercises include:

- **Sprint/walk.** No more walking at a constant pace for 45 minutes, which is time-consuming, boring, and short on results. You'll want to walk at a nice clip and then do your sprint, which might be only a really fast walk at first! If you live in an area with hills, a faster burst up a hill is a great way to up your intensity.

- **Do stationary cycling.** Go at a resistance level of 0–1 at 70 rpm, stand up, and then push the resistance level as high as possible while keeping the rpm over 100.

- **Go up and down stairs.** Walk or run up as many as you can in 30 seconds and then walk down and repeat. You can also take two steps at a time to mix it up.

- **Jump rope.** Jump as fast as you can for 30 seconds and then walk around to recover.

- **Use an X-iser.** This is my favorite no-excuses bursting machine. It is indestructible (my teen boys couldn't break it), lightweight, and portable (fits into your suitcase to take on an airplane) and is capable of kicking your butt, no matter your fitness level. This is the machine I have all of my VIP clients get. You stand on the machine with both knees slightly bent so that you always keep some pressure on your thighs (and they will scream, trust me on this) and then drive your heels down in a stepping motion as fast as possible for 30–60 seconds. When this gets easy, you can tighten the resistance and/or add some dumbbells to do overhead presses and biceps curls (while continuing to step) to make it even harder!

If You're Moderately Fit

Let's say you're someone who does a daily walk or moderate aerobic exercise for an hour three times a week. Decrease the time and add four to eight bursts. Start the bursting after the

Signs You Are Not Bursting Hard Enough

- You can call your friend and catch up while doing your cardio.
- You can concentrate on reading a book while bursting.
- You don't ever seem to sweat.
- You do more talking than working out at the gym.
- You do all your exercises sitting or lying down.
- You feel as if you could take a nap—while exercising!

first 3 minutes of low intensity and do another 3 minutes of low intensity at the end to incorporate your warm-up and cool-down. Be sure to reduce your intensity for a minute between bursting sets while continuing to move to allow recovery time. If you are really bursting hard, the way you are supposed to, you won't last more than a minute and you will need that easy recovery time in between to catch your breath and get the fire out of your legs and lungs!

Bursting and Weight Training Guide

On my program, you will burst train one day and weight train the next for six days a week. Six days a week may seem like a major time commitment, *but* the total time is probably less than many people's standard—and less effective—thrice-weekly workouts.

And if you do Pilates, yoga, or any other activities, they don't replace your bursting or weight training workouts on this plan. Think of them as beneficial "exercise extras." I always suggest that my clients buy a pedometer to remind them to move more during their daily life. Good ways to do this are to park some distance from your destination, take the stairs rather than the elevator, and so on. You want to move as much as possible, but those extras never take the place of your scheduled workouts.

Now Let's Pick Up the Weights

On your nonbursting days, you will retreat to your gym or home gym to pump it up! You must add this resistance training to sculpt your arms into beauties. Think of resistance training as the way to increase your "interest rate," as adding muscle means that your body will burn more calories all day long. Muscle is where we burn fat and become more sensitive to insulin, so adding muscle will help burn more fat calories while holding everything in tighter. Consider muscle mass as your fat-burning, metabolic-boosting "Spanx."

Remember, no little wimpy pink girlie weights. Leave them on your desk as paperweights. We're serious about creating perfect arms for you and thus you will need much heavier weights and to follow a few keys to muscle training. With weight training, as with bursting, go for intensity. I will have you focusing on multijoint, full-body movements. They also mimic movements we do in everyday life, so they will improve your activities of daily living while also reducing your risk of injury.

Some of the exercises that follow require your fitness ball. Now is the time to get it ready and learn how to keep it in optimal condition.

How to Prepare Your Fitness Ball

1. Remove it from the package and inspect it for shipping damage. It is normal for the ball to have slight fold marks. Spread the ball out on the floor with the hole open. If the ball feels cold or hot, let it come to room temperature before inflating it.

2. Inflate the ball according to the ball's maximum diameter/size (the height off the floor); do not inflate according to pressure. Inflate the ball by using one of the following methods:

   - A hand pump with a cone-shaped nozzle
   - An electric air compressor with a cone-shaped nozzle
   - Compressed air from the gas station

3. Test the ball periodically for comfort by sitting on it. Fill the ball until your knees and hips are at or above a 90-degree angle

4. Do not overinflate the ball. You should be able to push the ball inward roughly 2 inches when it is fully inflated.

General Maintenance

Common sense is always the rule.

1. Check for sharp objects on the floor before using your ball. Although a burst-resistant ball will not explode if punctured, it can tear and deflate.
2. Do not use the ball outdoors; this increases the risk of puncturing it. Keep the ball away from pets, who will think it's a toy!
3. Check the ball regularly for scratches, and wash it with warm soapy water.
4. Do not let the ball come into contact with materials printed with black ink.

Weight-Lifting Exercise Guide at a Glance

You will do 8 to 12 reps of the heaviest weight you can handle in good form. If you can get up to 12, increase the weight. If you can't get up to 8, lighten it. Take a 1-minute rest break between sets.

Every third week, you will do endurance sets to mix things up. For these sets, work at slightly below the weight you use for your 8 to 12 reps and continue to push through to 15 to 25 reps until you can't stand the "burn." Take a 1-to-2-minute break between sets.

Shake It Up

One of the techniques long used by top bodybuilders is muscle confusion. Just as with bursting, you don't want your body to adapt to what you are doing because then you won't continue to progress. As a countering measure, continue to change things up. You can do this by changing exercises, weights, sets, reps, and tempo. We will be shaking things up during this program by modifying sets and reps and by using a technique known as "supersetting." I have divided the upper-body exercises into two sections: upper-body pushing and upper-body pulling. Some of the weeks, you will work completely within one group—e.g., doing all upper-body pushing first—to totally fatigue those muscles before moving over to the other group. Other weeks you will alternate between two opposing exercises with shorter rest breaks; this again is "supersetting." An example would be alternating sets of push-ups with sets of pull-ups.

Pushing to Fatigue

As discussed, you will work in sets of 8 to 12 during most of the program. If you can get past 12 reps easily, you need to make your weights heavier because you're not pushing yourself to fatigue. Heavy it up! You're working to fatigue to create lactic acid, which then increases human growth hormone and builds muscle.

I can't tell you what your fatigue level will be, and it will change as your body becomes stronger. The general rule is that the workouts should *never* feel easy. The minute you start breezing through the workouts, increase the weights and work to fatigue again. This is about challenging yourself.

The Vanity Trio

Primarily, I teach my clients to focus on multijoint exercises, but there are also little sculpting exercises that isolate the vanity muscles: biceps, triceps, and shoulders. These exercises are not the focus but simply throw your program (and how you look in T-shirts and dresses) over the top. It's like putting a little bit of glittery cool eye shadow on at the end of a great makeup job or placing a perfect necklace over a gorgeous dress. You still have to lay the foundation with the multijoint, free weight exercises.

The Exercises

Upper-Body Pulling

Bent-over Row

Primary muscles worked: lats, back extensors, rhomboids, rear shoulders, biceps, core

- Stand with a slight bend at the knees, holding the weights at your sides.
- Lean over, extending your chest while reaching your hips back.
- Allow your arms to hang straight down toward the floor with your palms facing your thighs.
- Looking forward at the ground (not up), pull your elbows up and rotate your hands until your palms are nearly touching your upper rib cage, and your elbows point toward the ceiling.
- Lower the weights to the starting position with control. Repeat.

Tip: Keep your belly button pulled in toward your spine to engage your core and protect your lower back.

One-Arm Row with Ball

Primary muscles worked: lats, rhomboids, rear shoulders, biceps

- Place your feet just wider than shoulder width with an exercise ball directly in front of you.
- Begin by holding one weight in your right hand, hanging toward the floor.
- Keeping your back straight, lean on the ball with your left hand, your chest up and hips back.
- Looking forward, pull your elbow up and twist your hand until your palm touches your side, and your elbow points toward the ceiling.
- Lower the weight to the starting position with control.
- Repeat. Switch hands for the next set.

Tip: Keep your shoulders level and core strong. Do not twist your trunk during the movement.

Upright Row

Primary muscles worked: shoulders, upper back, biceps

- Stand with your feet shoulder width apart with the weights hanging down in front of your body, their ends touching.
- Raise your upper arms, leading with your elbows while bringing the weights up the front of your body as if you

were tracing an imaginary midpoint, stopping when your elbows become level with your shoulders.

- Lower the weights back to the starting position.

Tip: Keep your chin up and your belly button tucked in.

Upper-Body Pushing

Chest Press on Ball

Primary muscles worked: chest, front of shoulders, triceps

- Sit on a ball and walk out so that your head and shoulder blades are resting on the ball.
- Lift your hips by contracting your glute muscles to make a bridge. (Your feet should be shoulder width apart and below your knees to give you a stable support.)
- Bring the dumbbells to your shoulders. Then extend your arms over your chest and bring the dumbbells together to make a triangle over your chest.
- Lower the weights back to the starting position and repeat.

Tip: You will need to engage your core throughout the exercise to avoid falling off the ball.

Overhead Press on Ball

Primary muscles worked: shoulders, upper back, triceps

- Sit on an exercise ball with your belly button pulled toward the spine.
- Hold the weights in front of your shoulders, your palms facing in.
- Push the weights up until your arms are extended.
- When your arms are extended, they should be slightly in front of you rather than directly overhead.
- Lower the weights to the starting position and repeat.

Tip: Keep your chin lifted slightly and your core stable.

Dips off Chair

Primary muscles worked: triceps

- Sit tall on the edge of a chair, your palms flat and your fingers hanging over the edge.
- Keeping your shoulders and elbows behind you, gently scoot off the edge of the chair and lower your hips toward the floor until your elbows make a 90-degree angle.
- Push up against the chair to extend your elbows and lift your body back to the starting position.

Tip: Stay near the chair by keeping your hips angled back toward it. Your back should be perpendicular to the floor at all times. Lift your chest toward the ceiling to keep your back straight and your chin up. Tuck your elbows and arms in toward your body to prevent them from flaring out to the sides. To make this exercise easier, keep your legs bent. To increase the intensity, straighten your legs and/or put them up on a stability ball.

The Vanity Trio: Diagonal Raise, Biceps Curl on Ball, and French Press on Ball

These are optional exercises that will be done at the end of your workout. You can do them every time or add them in twice a week.

Diagonal Raise

Primary muscles worked: all three parts of the shoulder muscle

- Stand with your feet shoulder width apart and your knees slightly bent with your belly button pulled in toward your spine.
- Hold a dumbbell in your right hand and bring it to your left hipbone.
- Keeping your elbow slightly bent throughout the movement, lift the dumbbell diagonally outward so it ends up above your right shoulder and your elbow is level with your shoulder.
- Return to starting position and repeat.

Tip: Do not swing the weight or arch your back when you are raising the weight. Keep your elbow fixed with a slight bend throughout the movement.

Biceps Curl on Ball

Primary muscles worked: biceps

- With your head and upper torso resting on a ball, hold a dumbbell in each hand and walk out into the bridging position. Your hips are lifted, and your feet are shoulder width apart and below your knees.
- Lower and extend your arms to your sides, resting them against the ball. Lift the dumbbells to your shoulders.
- Return to starting position and repeat.

Tip: Keep your glute muscles contracted to keep your core stable during the exercise. Do not hyperextend your elbow joint during the movement.

French Press on Ball

Primary muscles worked: triceps

- Sit on a ball. Holding on to a dumbbell with both hands, extend both arms overhead. Your palms should be facing the ceiling, and your fingers should overlap.
- Lower the weight behind your head, bending your elbows just past a 90-degree angle.

- Return your arms back overhead.
- Return to starting position and repeat.

Tip: Be sure to keep your belly button pulled toward your spine to support your core and avoid arching your back.

Your Weight Training Schedule

Here's what you'll need to do each week.

- **Week 1:** Two sets of 8 to 12 reps of the heaviest weight you can handle with good form. Do your exercises in this order:

  - Chest Press on ball
  - Overhead Press on Ball
  - Dips off Chair
  - Bent-over Row
  - One-Arm Row with Ball
  - Upright Row
  - Vanity Trio (at least twice this week)

- **Week 2:** Superset: three sets of 8 to 12 reps of the heaviest weight you can handle with good form. Alternate sets of each exercise. For example: do one set of Bent-over Row, then one set of Chest Press on Ball, and repeat.

- Bent-over Row and Chest Press on Ball

- One-Arm Row and Dips off Chair

- Overhead Press on Ball and Upright Row

- Vanity Trio (at least twice this week): Superset of Biceps Curls on Ball and French Press on Ball

- **Week 3:** Two sets to fatigue. You should do 15 to 25 reps and feel a bit more of a "burn." Do your exercises in this order:

  - Bent-over Row

  - One-Arm Row with ball

  - Upright Row

  - Chest Press on Ball

  - Overhead Press on Ball

  - Dips off Chair

  - Vanity Trio (at least twice this week)

- **Week 4:** Three sets of 8 to 12 reps of the heaviest weight you can handle with good form. Do your exercises in this order:

  - Chest Press on Ball

  - Overhead Press on Ball

  - Dips off Chair

  - Bent-over Row

  - One-Arm Row with Ball

- Upright Row
- Vanity Trio (at least twice this week)

- **Week 5:** Three sets of 8 to 12 reps of the heaviest weight you can handle with good form.

  - Repeat the supersets from week 2
  - Vanity Trio (at least twice this week): superset of Biceps Curl on Ball and French Press on Ball

- **Week 6:** Three sets to fatigue. You should do 15 to 25 reps until you feel the "burn." Do your exercises in this order:

  - Bent-over Row
  - One-Arm Row with Ball
  - Upright Row
  - Chest Press on Ball
  - Overhead Press on Ball
  - Dips off Chair
  - Vanity Trio (at least twice this week)

A few final Words on Exercise

- Find a friend to do the program with you. This will keep you accountable and make it more fun, and you can challenge each other. Be sure to check each other's form.

- Change your bursting activities to keep your body from getting set on one type of exercise and to prevent boredom. Keep your body guessing!

- While exercising, make sure to listen to your body. If you have pain in your joints or soreness to the touch or discomfort that lasts more than two days, your body is telling you to back down.

- If a mirror is available, it's helpful to do your exercises in front of one and watch your form. This is focused time.

- If you're sore, don't mask the pain with over-the-counter drugs such as ibuprofen. When you take away your ability to feel pain, you can really hurt yourself. Listen to your body, and don't cover up symptoms that are telling you to rest.

- Remember that recovery and rest are just as important as your workouts. Just stay committed and focused if you need to take an extra day off. You're not slacking off but listening to your body.

- After a workout, take a hot bath with 1 or 2 cups of Epsom salts added to the water. It feels wonderful, it may help reduce muscle soreness, and you earned it!

5. Grow 'Em

If I could sit down with you right now and share the best prescription for health, I would flip right to this chapter and read it to you because it focuses on two major changes you can vow to make today that will continue to pay you health dividends for the rest of your life. Two of the best-kept secrets when it comes to wellness and weight loss come from areas that seem so simple but are often ignored: sleep and stress.

Sleep

Let's start with sleep because most women have such busy days with work, family, and their homes that sleep is an afterthought.

If something has to give, it's usually a good eight hours of slumber. Maybe you sleep five or six hours one night and then get only four the next because you have a big report due. You stay up until midnight working on the computer and then can't get to sleep until 2 A.M. The following morning, you walk around in a tired haze, but a few cups of coffee during the day give you enough of a jolt to do what's necessary before you struggle to capture a few zzzzs again.

You need to stop living this sleep-deprived lifestyle right now and focus on making high-quality sleep a priority for several reasons, including long-term health and success on this program. Maybe you're saying, "I don't need that much sleep. Five hours is all I've ever needed, and it has been this way since high school." I still beg to differ and ask you to do what I suggest on these next pages because it will completely change your body, your energy level, and your life.

Studies show that a healthy lifestyle should include not only healthy eating habits and adequate amounts of physical activity but also an optimal amount of sleep. When you get good-quality sleep, your body has time to rebuild your muscles, which is mandatory in this program and for optimal health. Sleep is an *active* process that provides rejuvenating functions for the entire body, including muscle growth, tissue repair, and even emotional processing.

Think of sleep as a time not just of rest but also of restoration. It's when your body and mind recalibrate for the next day.

Did you know that it's nearly impossible to lose weight without proper sleep? And that's not the only serious pitfall of not connecting with your pillow and blanket for enough time and at the right times.

A study from the University of Chicago showed that even when people eat properly and exercise on a regular basis, if they get less than the recommended seven to nine hours of sleep per night, they are at a greater risk of obesity. Why? It creates hormonal chaos in your body and elevates your stress hormones while your appetite soars and your energy level plummets. Lack of sleep also makes you a better fat storer, especially in the belly area. And it impairs your ability to build muscle.

Let's go back to the science of your body. Consider that a single night of sleep deprivation increases ghrelin levels and feelings of hunger in normal-weight, healthy men and women. It also decreases insulin sensitivity, meaning your body can't "hear" insulin's message as well and thus secretes more. A higher level of insulin at a fasting level can shut down fat burning. If you sleep less, you will eat more and in turn put on weight. It's that simple.

The end result of being tired all the time is that you're going to look for "quick pick-me-ups" that temporarily boost your energy, such as caffeine and sugar. Now you're caught in a vicious cycle.

You're exhausted, so you gulp caffeine and sugar; an hour later you feel crappy, and then you crash. What do you do now? You chug *more* caffeine and sugar and go through another unhealthy cycle that might induce insomnia when you desperately try to recharge at night. For many people, this is their daily existence.

Sleep is especially crucial when you're exercising because sleep time is when your body produces more human growth hormone. That's the "juice" that some celebs pay well over a thousand dollars a month to inject into their system because it keeps their bodies young. If you can get this boost for free by doing something as wonderful as sleeping, why not make sure you're rewarding your body by just closing your eyes and drifting away?

Let me reemphasize that sleep is when your body repairs and rebuilds your muscles. If you're not sleeping well, you're not accomplishing this all-important restorative action. *When it comes to building muscle, the repair time is just as important as the time you spend exercising.*

By the way, here's more encouragement: if you don't sleep enough you're also in danger of losing your sex drive and aging faster. Without naming names, think of the young movie stars who "party all night." Ever notice how five minutes ago they looked their real age—in their early twenties—and suddenly they appear to be about forty? It seems to happen overnight. Why? Their bodies hardly ever get the restorative sleep necessary to keep them looking young and beautiful.

armed and dangerous

Even one less hour of sleep per night than the ideal will impact your entire life and will derail any weight loss or muscle-building exercise program.

A Case Study

Consider the case of Susan,* a client of mine who followed her workout plan and ate three healthful meals daily, as I've outlined to you in the previous chapters. About halfway through her program, she hit a major plateau and stopped losing weight. Her goal of getting into a little strappy dress for her sister's wedding seemed to stall.

We checked her journal to make sure she was challenging herself with her muscle workouts and cardio blasting while eating the right foods at the right time in perfect quantities. Susan was also trying to revamp her business and was burning the midnight oil. She was sleeping about four to five hours a night and then waking up at 5 A.M. to work out. She didn't really feel tired because she had always operated on too little sleep. No one had ever linked the extra 30 pounds she had kept on for the past decade to her sleep habits.

* The anecdotes about clients are composites and do not represent any actual particular person.

When I told Susan that she was suffering from chronic sleep deprivation, she shook her head as if it couldn't be true. "How could I run a business and take care of my five-year-old if I was chronically sleep-deprived?" she asked.

Then I asked her to do something that sounded crazy to her at first: make sure she got a solid 7 to 9 hours a night of unbroken sleep that would allow her body to achieve all the stages of rejuvenating slumber. Two weeks later, the weight started coming off again and she quickly attained her body-weight goal while marveling at the amazing new energy she had to use for her family and her business. And that little black dress looked fabulous on her.

How do you know if you're getting enough sleep? Try my simple sleep quiz to see if you're chronically sleep-deprived.

JJ's Sleep Quiz

Answer each of the following questions with a "yes" if it applies to you more than one night a week:

- Does it take you thirty minutes or more to fall asleep at night?
- Do you sleep less than seven to nine hours a night?
- Do you get out of bed once or more during the night?
- Are you aware of waking up two or more times during the night?

Bent-over Row (p. 100)

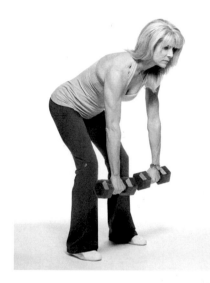

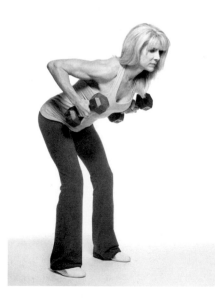

LESLEY BOHM

One-Arm Row with Ball (p. 101)

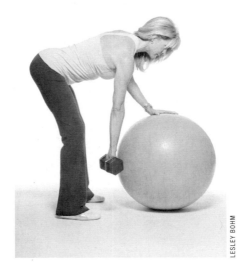

LESLEY BOHM

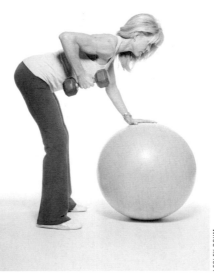

LESLEY BOHM

Upright Row (p. 101)

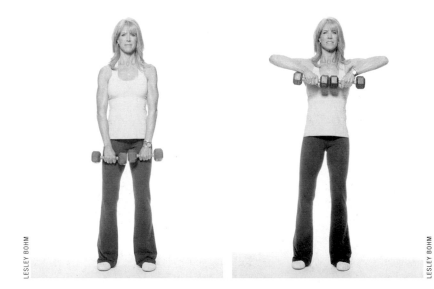

LESLEY BOHM

LESLEY BOHM

Chest Press on Ball (p. 102)

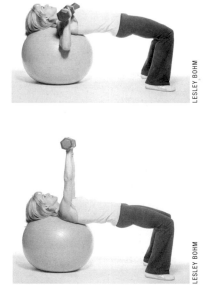

LESLEY BOHM

LESLEY BOHM

Overhead Press on Ball (p. 103)

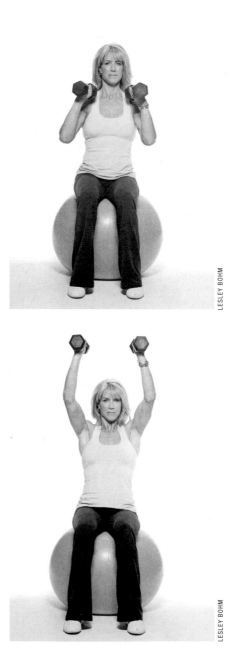

LESLEY BOHM

LESLEY BOHM

Dips off chair—Beginner (p. 103)

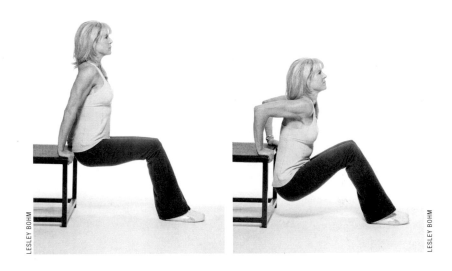

Dips off chair—Advanced (p. 103)

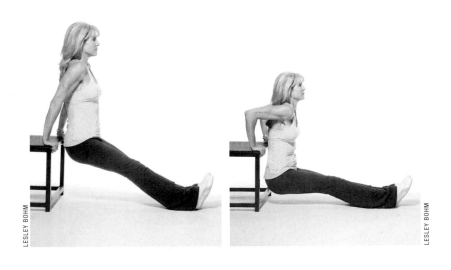

Diagonal Raise (p. 104)

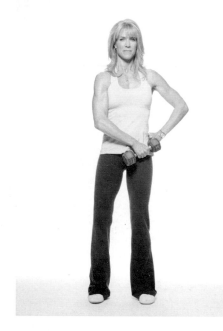

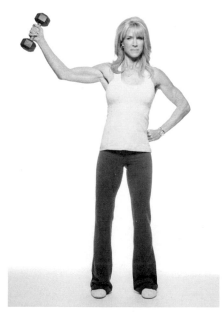

Biceps Curl on Ball (p. 105)

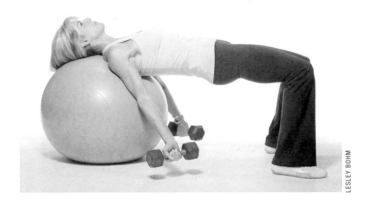

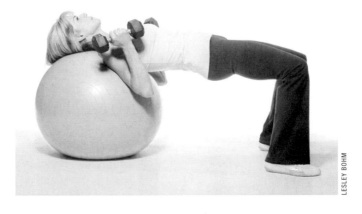

French Press on Ball (p. 105)

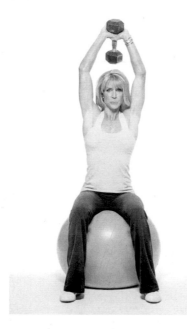

LESLEY BOHM

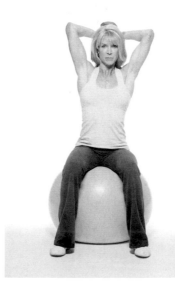

LESLEY BOHM

- Does your partner tell you that you snore or toss and turn a lot?
- Do you sleep in a room with any disturbances, including light or noise?
- Do you feel groggy when you wake up and struggle to "turn your brain on"?
- Do you need an alarm clock to wake up?
- Do you go to bed later than 11 P.M.?
- Do you get up earlier than 6 A.M.?
- Do you vary the time you wake up in the morning by more than 30 minutes?
- Do you use medications (over-the-counter or prescription) to sleep?
- Do you feel sleepy during the day, especially between 1 and 3 P.M.?

Count up all of your "yes" answers. Guess what? Even one "yes" indicates less-than-optimal sleep patterns and can set you up for health problems.

armed and dangerous

Even one night of bad sleep (lack of it or sleep that's interrupted) will make you less insulin sensitive and your cortisol and adrenaline levels will be higher than normal. The net effect of this is increased appetite, poor fat burning, more fat storing around your waist, and a higher set point for being able to burn it off.

JJ's Sleeping Checklist

Now that you know the pitfalls of not getting enough sleep, it's time to discuss what you need to do—starting tonight—to correct the situation. It's easy, and your body will respond almost immediately. Here's your action plan:

- You need to sleep seven to nine uninterrupted hours each night during the normal sleep cycle, which is between 9 P.M. and 7 A.M. This is the way human beings were meant to sleep to restore their bodies through the natural circadian rhythm. This way your body will go through all the proper sleep phases.
- No more naps! I'm not a fan of catnaps because they throw off your circadian rhythm. I always feel confused and not at all refreshed after a nap. If you must take a nap, take just one early in the day, but I'd rather you pass on it. You really want to be tired enough to get your proper sleep at night and go through those sleep phases.

- Cool it on the caffeine. Limit it to one to two cups in the morning only. Did you know caffeine has a twelve-hour half-life, so the coffee you have at breakfast is still in your system in the evening? Now imagine if you have a cup of coffee after dinner. Hello, insomnia.

- Remember that there is no eating after your healthful dinner, which should be three hours before bedtime. You shouldn't be hungry or uncomfortably full when you get into bed.

- Set an alarm *at night* for an hour before bedtime to alert you when it's time to wind down for the day. This is a time to let your brain relax and to refrain from stimulating activities, so your body will get ready for sleep. Do not work on the computer, watch a violent TV show, fret over the horrible state of the economy, or have a heated talk on the phone. Instead, sip some herbal tea, take a hot bath with lavender in it, dim the lights, cool down your bedroom, or read a book. Just relax. You're in wind-down mode now. If you're in a relationship, be sure your partner respects this pattern and, hopefully, joins you.

- Create a lovely bedroom with a comfortable bed and make sure the room is completely dark so your pineal gland will be able to convert serotonin to melatonin, the hormone that helps you sleep. This means don't fall asleep with the TV on. In fact, I strongly recommend removing it from your bedroom.

- Don't bring work to bed. No laptops under the covers. Your bed is for sleeping and romance. Period!

- Wake up at the same time every day no matter what time you fall asleep. Your body will welcome and get used to this sleep routine.

armed and dangerous

Every hour of sleep counts. People who get only five hours of sleep a night are 50 percent more likely to be obese. Even those who manage to sleep six hours a night are 23 percent more likely to be obese!

Don't Break Up Your Sleep

Catnaps are out as a way to achieve proper sleep, but now I want to explain why you can't break up your sleep into two or more cycles a day. Sleep *quality* is as important as sleep *quantity*. The quality of your sleep depends on your time in restorative slumber, including REM and deep-sleep phases. Over the course of the night, you typically go through four to five sleep cycles (a typical cycle lasts 90 to 110 minutes), with deep sleep in the earlier cycles and REM sleep in the later cycles. Your goal is to go through *all* of the cycles because the REM phase affects learning and memory while the deep-sleep periods impact growth hormone release, rest, and recovery while strengthening your immune system. Your body needs to go through all these phases, so please sleep in one long, uninterrupted period.

During this solid type of sleep, you will not wake up to do

other activities, including going to the bathroom. You need to stop that right now because it's probably just a habit and not necessary to healthy bladder function. If you do get up in the middle of the night to use the bathroom, evaluate your fluid intake during the last few hours before you get into bed.

Some workaholic types get up in the middle of the night to check their email or flip on the tube for a few minutes. Stop! You don't want to break your sleep cycle with stimulating activities that will make it hard for you to fall back asleep because now you've fired up your neurons and your brain is racing. Practice self-control—stay off the phone, TV, and computer once you have powered down for the night.

A lot of my friends are creative people who proudly say that they're "night owls." They get their big ideas and inspirations when the sun goes down and often work late into the night. It's time to rearrange your schedule, and I promise your creativity won't suffer. Night owls should start by backing up their bedtime by thirty minutes every few days. Let's say you naturally go to bed at 1 A.M. Try 12:30 A.M. Every few days, back it up another thirty minutes until you're going to bed earlier and it feels natural. Wake up between 6 and 8 A.M. each morning, flip on the lights, and even play some heart-pounding music. This is a great time for night owls to exercise and do their bursting sets. You are changing your patterns to be awake during the day (no more sleeping until noon) and going to bed earlier. The transition

> ## Avoid These Common Sleep Stealers
>
> - Unresolved health issues
> - Anxiety and stress
> - Disruptive bedroom environment
> - Inconsistent sleep schedule
> - Stimulating nighttime activities
> - Poor diet
> - Disruptive bedmates (kids, pets, snoring spouse)

might take a few weeks, but I promise you will be thrilled with the results.

Sleep Cheat Sheet

Please remember this:

- Adults need 7 to 9 hours of sleep per night, with the average need being 8¼ hours. If you are under a lot of stress, you will need more sleep.
- Light and dark dictate the normal circadian rhythm of the wake-and-sleep cycle. You need to rest when it's dark and be active when it's light.

- If you overstimulate yourself to stay up later at night, you will disrupt these sleep patterns.

- Don't believe the myth that you need to sleep less as you age. You need just as much sleep when you are older as you did when you were young.

- Remember that just because you're not tired in the morning doesn't mean you're getting enough sleep. If you run on stress hormones, you will have a false sense of energy. This can go on for many years until you crash and burn out.

- Don't drink caffeine after noon. Avoid sugar and refined carbs, which can cause nighttime hypoglycemia.

- Eat enough food during the day to avoid being hungry at bedtime, which can raise your stress hormones and make it hard to fall asleep and stay asleep.

- Limit or eliminate alcohol. Alcohol's hypoglycemic effects often cause you to wake up between 2 and 4 A.M.

- Quit smoking once and for all. Nicotine mimics the effects of adrenaline and affects sleep.

Stress

Is stress making your arms chunky and your waistline expand? These are just two of the evil effects that chronic stress can have on your body. Stress has several additional devastating affects on your health that are too numerous to list in this book, including accelerating aging and knocking out your sex drive. Stressing less is something you need to focus on for your overall health and sanity.

Since we're focusing on muscle building and fat loss, it's time to mention that stress can change the "set point" at which your body burns off fat and can increase fat storage, especially around your waistline.

Let's add it up: stress makes you old and fat, and it forces you to reach for a granny gown instead of a sexy nightie!

How does all of this happen? When you're under stress, your body mobilizes all your energy so you can survive the attack on your system. Our bodies are designed to do this in a short-term way during periods of unrest. The problem is that our modern lifestyle keeps us in a constant state of stress in which we work longer, sleep less, and have so many upheavals during the average day that we live in a stressed-out state. We're also dealing with artificial lighting, cell phones, and computers that constantly blink, buzz, light up, and keep us in a mild frenzy. It feels normal, but your body was not meant to deal with long-term stress. It's actually very dangerous to your health.

Do you feel as though you're always fighting through stressful moments that only lead to further on-the-edge situations? Your body is feeling the harried state and responds by breaking down muscle (mobilizing energy) and dumping it into the bloodstream as sugar. Wonder why so many Americans have a high fasting blood sugar level? When your body does this, it follows by raising your fat-storing hormone, insulin, to move the blood sugar into your cells. At this point, you will experience low blood sugar and will want some refined carbs and/or sugar to get your energy level up again (at least for a little while).

Stress can lead to both insulin and leptin resistance. Leptin is a hormone that is key in appetite regulation. If you become resistant to it due to stress, your body fat may increase because the leptin won't reduce your appetite and you will be hungry all of the time and probably gravitate to the kitchen. All the stress hormones are packing on the pounds, especially around the waistline, while making it harder to burn off the fat that's already there.

Finally, chronic stress can lower the production of other hormones, including testosterone and DHEA, that help burn fat, build muscle, and promote a healthy sex drive. In order for the body to keep pushing out cortisol to keep up with the stress demands, it steals it away from the other hormones. Stress can also impact your ability to create active thyroid hormone, which is one of the master controllers of your metabolism.

Chronic stress can lead to fatigue, PMS, anxiety, depression, obesity, and immune dysfunction. If you continue to live under chronic stress, eventually you will just burn out and feel exhausted all of the time even when you finally get some rest. This is your body's later-stage reaction to stress, which is to conserve energy and go into "famine physiology." This is when it feels as if nothing you do to lose weight or build muscle seems to work. And if you do overexercise and cut your calorie intake drastically, you can actually make yourself worse.

Here's why. Let's say you go on a diet by cutting calories and plan to lose weight. Your body instantly blocks you because it believes the calorie cutting is just another stressful event that it must cope with in order to survive. What to do? Why not slow down your metabolism? Unfortunately, at the same time, your body lowers your immune system and accelerates the aging process.

I don't mean to stress you out further; I simply want you to recognize that you must work on getting all the unnecessary stresses out of your life—and you need to start right now.

armed and dangerous

Moisturize all you want! Stress accelerates your rate of cellular aging. If you want to feel and look younger, make a conscious effort to get as much stress out of your life as possible.

Is Stress Making Your Arms Fat?

Answer "yes" or "no" to the following questions. Count your "no" answers after you complete Part A. Count your "yes" answers after completing Part B.

Part A: Stress Relievers

- Do you have a close support network of family and friends?
- Do you have a spiritual foundation from which you draw strength and faith?
- Do you feel that you have control over your life and its direction?
- Are you happy in your career or job?
- Do you do burst-style exercise regularly three times per week?
- Do you eat three meals per day at least six days of the week?
- Do you take downtime each day to experience your own personal bliss?
- Are you comfortable financially?
- Do you keep your weight within your ideal weight range and body fat composition?
- Do you regularly get seven to nine hours of quality sleep per night?

Total number of "no" answers is _____.

Part B: Stress Provokers and Indicators

- Do you regularly consume caffeine, alcohol, and/or sugar and refined carbohydrates?
- Do you frequently feel fearful and/or that things are beyond your control?
- Do you struggle to remember things?

- Do you suffer from allergies, chronic fatigue, fibromyalgia, asthma, or headaches?
- Do you suffer from digestive problems, including heartburn, gas, bloating, diarrhea, or constipation?
- Do you engage in endurance training (cardio exercise for forty-five-plus minutes a day, three or more times a week)?
- Does it take you thirty minutes or longer to fall asleep at night? Do you have difficulty sleeping through the night?
- Are you sensitive to smells?
- Have you lost interest in sex?
- Are you more tired after you work out?
- Are you impatient or easily irritated?
- Have you experienced any major life stressor (positive or negative) in the past year (i.e., death of a loved one, major illness, divorce, marriage, birth of a child, move, change of job, financial change)?
- Do you need caffeine to wake you up in the morning or help you make it through the day?
- Do you get sick three or more times a year?
- Do you crave carbohydrates or sugary foods? Do you crave salty foods?

Total number of "yes" answers is _____.

Grand total: _____

If you scored three or more in either part or four or more overall, you need to address your stress! Ideally, no matter what you scored, you will want to rectify any "no" answers in Part A and "yes" answers in Part B. Of course, you can tackle only what's possible to change, but you can focus on short- and long-term strategies to correct those stressful life areas because now you know they're a big detriment to your health and metabolism.

Just remember one of my favorite quotes from Dr. Hans Selye: "Adopting the right attitude can convert a negative stress into a positive one."

You should also be aware that there is good stress, such as when we fall in love, get married, retire, have a baby, buy a house, or get promoted. Then there is bad stress, such as when a spouse dies, we have a bad fight with a significant other, we get divorced, we lose our job, we change occupation, or we have a serious illness. When you're forced to navigate times of bad stress, pay close attention to taking better care of yourself and practicing destressing techniques. Remember, a large part of stress is your perception of it and reaction to it. Ensure that you are adequately armed with the tactics from Part A to help you cope better.

Are These Poor Lifestyle Habits Stressing You Out?

Here are some activities that are very stressful on the body that you can fix quickly to lower your stress:

- Excessive intake of caffeine (more than one to two servings daily)
- Excessive intake of alcohol (more than one serving daily)
- A very-low-carb diet
- Skipping meals
- Sugar
- Nicotine
- Endurance training
- Sleep deprivation

How Else Can I Destress?

We live in a world where it's impossible to remove all stresses from our lives. Your job is to eliminate as many stresses as you can and avoid adding additional stresses if you can help it. You can also focus on how you perceive a situation and remind yourself a hundred times a day if necessary: don't sweat the small stuff, and it's *all* small stuff!

There are ways that all of us can destress. Why don't you try these?

- Sit down and really look at your schedule. Get rid of the activities that aren't necessary. Yes, you're still a nice person, but you won't be attending four charity events this month, and little Bobby won't be involved in five after-school activities. Practice saying "no" to events that aren't necessary and mean it.

- Try to bump people you find tough to deal with out of your life, if possible.

- Schedule a little bit of R&R time into every single day. I don't care if you spend ten minutes in a tub or read a chapter of a great new novel. This is time just for you, and nothing will interrupt it. Make sure to plan something *you* love to do at least once a week. You're not doing it for the kids or your mate. Take that time, and do what makes you happy.

- Research stress-busting techniques such as meditation and deep breathing in a book or on the Internet. Find one that works for you, and use it during especially trying moments.

- Never miss a workout, which, I will repeat again and again, is one of the best destressors in the world.

JJ's Favorite Ways to Knock Out Stress

- Put on your MP3 player or stereo and crank it up. Listen to your favorite songs.

- Read a great book that inspires you.
- Meditate and pray.
- Soak in a sudsy hot bathtub. Dim the lights in the bathroom. Light a candle, and put a DO NOT DARE DISTURB ME sign on the door.
- Read a magazine or a light novel.
- Watch a great comedy DVD.
- Take a walk in the woods.
- Play with your dog or cats. Animals have a great relaxing effect on human beings.
- Hold hands with or kiss your honey.
- Go window-shopping.
- Treat yourself to a fabulous spa treatment.
- Get out some paper and write, draw, or paint. It's doesn't have to be a masterpiece. Just explore the fun of doing something creative.
- Do your burst training. It will help your body deal with stress and instantly shut off the rest of your life.

armed and dangerous

Studies show that people who engage in regular physical activity are the most resistant to stress.

Now that you're sleeping better and getting some of the stress out of your life, you're feeling better than ever. It's important to revisit your motivation, because this is the time when many people slip up.

6. Don't Blow 'Em

You might think that this is the rah-rah chapter, where I give you motivational sayings to paste to your forehead or mantras to chant at night. *I won't blow it . . . I won't eat it . . . I will do my bursting to blast fat in the morning. Amen.* You've been working hard for several weeks, and now you're actually seeing wonderful results. Your arms are firmer and sleeker, and suddenly there is a thought floating through your mind that hasn't surfaced in years—or forever: *I might go for a cap sleeve or wear that sleeveless dress because my arms are looking . . . pretty good!*

No, this arm nirvana is not a dream but the reality of looking at your naked, more muscular, yet thinner sculpted limbs in the mirror. It's your Michelle Obama moment. Yes, you can—and did!

A funny thing happens to many of us on the road to success. We're used to thinking that we might screw it up now and throw just a bit of caution to the proverbial wind. Maybe you've done that with every other plan you've ever been on. I know a woman who dropped 100 pounds by following a strict diet plan for a year. Once she reached her goal, she suddenly paid attention to her grumbling tummy, acknowledged that she was starving, and accepted that her body was in the kind of famine mode she couldn't ignore anymore. Soon she started reaching for carbs, and eventually she gained back 50 pounds. Now she laments that she screwed up and blew it.

You're not going to *ever* do that on my watch.

You don't need sayings and mantras for a reason.

Why?

We're not approaching this program as a short-term change where you're on it one moment, succeeding and thriving, and off it the next one, blowing it and feeling mad and upset with yourself. If you approach this book as something that will change your life, you won't ever be in a situation where you worry about "blowing it." It just isn't a possibility.

I know that's a very different mind-set for most people who are used to going on temporary-fix diets or throwing themselves with gusto into the exercise trend of the week. Yes, you've counted points until you turned blue and then kickboxed your way into back spasms. You went on the plans, saw a few results, and then wandered away because while they were fun to visit, you really didn't want to live there.

When you approach something as if it were a short-term plan, you will have a short-term commitment to it.

But if you approach this book as a series of action steps to build lifelong habits that will totally transform your life once and for all, you will mentally be in a much different place. This mind-set shift makes *all* the difference.

You will not say, "This is how I eat and exercise for just six weeks."

You will say, "This is how I eat and exercise now, tomorrow, and forever."

Period.

Why You Gained It All Back Before

Let me zap you out of the diet mentality. On this plan, you're changing your metabolism and the way you burn calories because you're burning fat and not muscle. If you don't do that, for the rest of your life you're doomed to live the same diet dilemma where you lose a few pounds, only to gain them again. You end up feeling like a loser.

Let's say you're on a very restricted calorie plan and you're severely limiting your food intake on some diet from Hell. You might lose a few pounds or even many pounds over a period of time, but soon they start creeping back on. It's not your fault, because it's almost impossible for you to live resisting food. It gets boring, and your entire focus in life becomes when can you eat next and what can you eat.

You're focused on putting something into your stomach because you're honestly so hungry and not thinking about nutrition. Perhaps you're counting points and your entire universe now centers on "doing the math" for every bite of food. By the way, your body handles different foods in various ways, so you can't say that diet desserts, chicken, and an avocado all have the same "points" and you will lose weight from eating a certain amount of calories or points and have great arms and great energy. Weight loss depends on what, when, and how much you eat, how much and how you move, how you handle stress, and how well you sleep. You can't pick and choose the parts of the program that you want to follow and expect success.

This brings me back to why you may feel that you "failed" in the past. You continue to cut calories to the point where you're very hungry and your body can't maintain itself on such a small amount of food. You begin to eat more, and the pounds come back while your self-esteem sinks. You feel like a failure (again). This isn't your fault.

As human beings, we're hardwired to survive famines. The more food you cut out of your life, the more your body slows down the burning of fat and fuel in order to survive. Your body will conserve fat and increase stress hormones. In other words, you're working against your real goals while torturing yourself.

The saddest part of these diets is what they can do to your emotional and physical health. First, they make you feel like a loser, and then something even worse happens to so-called yo-yo dieters.

You go on the next restrictive caloric plan and lose more muscle than fat (again). But when you gain the weight back, you pack on more fat than muscle. Gradually, you become fluffier and fluffier as your metabolism slows down even more over a period of time and ten more silly plans. You might lose another 20 pounds and then gain back 20 of fat, while you lose even more muscle.

Fast weight loss done through extreme caloric restriction and lack of or the wrong type of exercise means that some of the weight you will lose is muscle. This is bad, as muscle is what drives our metabolism and where we burn fat. Worse yet, when you gain the weight back, you gain mainly fat weight. This vicious cycle goes on and on as you become fluffier and fluffier, fatter and fatter.

My plan is different because I'm shifting you away from the crazy concept that your body is a bank account and that in order to lose weight you have to severely reduce your calorie intake and burn as many calories as possible throughout the day and toward understanding that your body is a chemistry lab. Yes, calories do count, but where they come from counts more. Yes, you want to move more, but you want to make sure that when you exercise it is focused, high-quality movement that will turn your body into a lean, fat-burning machine.

Okay, JJ, So What Happens If I . . .

You wake up late one morning because the alarm didn't go off. Racing through your house, you barely splash three drops of water on yourself in the shower and then throw on some clothes. Breakfast? Oh shoot, you forgot about it. By 10 A.M. you're starving, but you also forgot your emergency foods, which are sitting on the counter where you left them last night before the frenzy of this morning. Without your apple or nuts, you wander into the kitchen at work and see a tray of half-dried-out doughnuts from the morning. You're so hungry that you grab one, thinking, This is the day from Hell and I'm going to just do what I need to do.

An hour later, you sit at your desk thinking Great, not only is my hair one big frizzy mess because I didn't dry it, but now I've blown my new plan by eating sugar and carbs. Loser, loser, loser.

Stop in the name of your health — both mental and physical!

This is not a derailment of your plan; it's an opportunity to reframe the way you're thinking. The "loser" stuff is putting you into the traditional diet mind-set: "I'm on a plan. I'm not on a plan. I'm having a good day. I'm having a bad day."

With my plan, there are no good days or bad days. You're simply learning to cope with a new way of life while being extraconscious about replacing bad habits with new ones that are compatible with your new lifestyle. You're not having a bad day. You're simply going to work on living in a way that supports having great energy, great arms, great health, and great form, plus fosters a healthy immune system, strong bones, and a clear mind. (Hey, if those goals aren't worth shooting for, I don't know which ones are!)

Sure, there will be times when you might slip up. That's okay. I repeat: it's okay. Don't beat yourself up!

You just want to ask yourself after the slip: "How can I change my life to support me in being successful?"

Backtracking after a Slip

So you ate half a pizza with the girls. You wolfed down a dozen chocolate chip cookies. You blew off exercise tonight because you really wanted to watch a show on TV. There will be times like these, but use them as a tool. Ask yourself how you can handle the situation next time so that you win. By the way, it may mean not putting yourself into the situation in the first place!

Your task is to break this down to the simplest facts. Perhaps you went to a party where you ate too much pizza, and now you know it was the situation that created the problem. Maybe you forgot to carry your picture with your head on someone else's body as your security blanket. Perhaps you pigged out at lunch because you skipped breakfast.

Facts and information will make you successful in the long run. Think back to where the problem started in the first place, so you can keep it from happening again. Now you're armed with some powerful tools. Next time, you will make sure you have plenty of those pictures in your purse. You will set the alarm fifteen minutes early, so you never miss breakfast. You will remember to eat before a party because then you won't be so tempted to dive into anything that's dubbed "deep dish." Instead of regret, you've just deepened your commitment to your new lifestyle and to troubleshooting all the roadblocks in your way.

Return to Your Goals

I believe that if you can think of something, you can see it—and then it happens. Your success needs to be in the forefront of your mind. Your belief has to be strong, and it must be unwavering. If you truly believe that you can be a healthy, lean person, you will stay in that place mentally (think it), see it (with your picture), and then make it happen (following my plan).

If you're not so sure that you will be successful (you're not really thinking it), then you really can't see it and it probably won't come true.

I'm unwavering in my positive thinking that I will live as a strong, lean, healthy person. This isn't an option but a fact. My mind stays there. When I want to reach for a piece of cake, my conviction is so strong that I won't allow some gloppy, sugary, not-even-that-tasty mush of sugar, water, and waxy fake frosting mess with my dreams of who I am.

If it's situations that cause your slips, reevaluate how you deal with them. Did you practice the three-bite rule? Did you avoid happy hour? Did you go to a cocktail party at dinnertime when you were starving and those little puffed pastry things were the closest things to food you could find? Deep-fried chicken coated with bread crumbs dipped in sweet-and-sour sauce is not something that's going to help you in the long run. It's a little protein covered by carbs and fat served with a sugary sauce, which in reality makes it more like dessert.

Ask yourself, "What can I do to make this easy on myself?"

Life should not be hard. I wouldn't bring Starbucks Java Chip ice cream into my house as a mental test or to see if I can really take three bites today and then leave it alone for the next week. I don't want to make my life that hard. Successful people remove obstacles and don't put them in their path on purpose. What is the point of making your life tougher when the world does a good job of that all by itself? Be kind to yourself, and make your days easier.

The more you work on this way of being nice to yourself, the easier it will become for you until it's just second nature and you don't even think about it anymore.

Replace Old Thinking with New Thinking

To prevent self-defeat, here's the new thought process in action.

The Old You: I'm on a diet, but my craving for pizza was so strong I sneaked over to a restaurant with the word "Hut" in it and ordered a medium just for myself. Now my stomach is bloated. I don't feel good, and I'm a total failure. Plus, I probably just gained three pounds, and since it's already a bad diet day, I might as well stop at Dairy Queen on the way home. If I'm going to blow it, I might as well really blow it.

The New You: I'm on a life-changing plan; having a few slices of pizza doesn't mean I failed. I will just get back on the horse right now and go immediately back to my plan for success. I won't eat ten other bad things because now it's a "bad day." There are no bad days. I just slipped. How did it happen? Oh, right, I didn't have breakfast this morning, and I was starving and not in the right framework mentally to make good food choices. Next time I will eat breakfast and have a salad for lunch. Or, if I am really craving a pizza, I will go to one of the gourmet pizza restaurants with a friend or two and share a thin-crust veggie pizza and a great salad.

The Old You: I've been exercising so hard every day for three weeks, and now it's a cold, rainy night and I just don't feel like it. How can skipping one day hurt me? Wait, maybe I skipped a day last week, too. Screw it. It's Friday, and I'll get back on my plan on Monday—I hope.

The New You: I've made appointments with myself and scheduled exercise sessions in the mornings because it's cold at night, and let's be honest about one thing: I've already done five sessions this week and that's good. I did miss tonight, but I will start again tomorrow. It doesn't take that much time to exercise right, and I can always find time to fit it in.

The Old You: I've been good all week, and now I'm going to a backyard barbecue at my neighbor's house. I've saved up for this event, and I'm going to go hog wild and eat ribs and potato salad and then have the homemade peach pie for dessert. You have to enjoy life, and I'm really going for it!

The New You: I've been on my plan and feeling stronger all week, plus I think I went down another clothing size. I'm going to wear the strappy blue sundress that I can't believe now fits and great heels because I'm going to that backyard barbecue down the street to have fun and see friends. But I'm going to be smart about it. I'm bringing a huge cut-up raw veggie tray with the best homemade salsa and side of hummus from a local Greek restaurant. I'm staying away from the chips and all that potato salad that's full of mayo. I'm going to have a bit of grilled chicken, and I know they'll have fresh fruit. They always have great wine, and I'll have a glass. Sure, Mary will be pushing the pie, but I'll just use the three-bite rule because it is pretty irresistible. Then I'll put my fork down and remember I'm really there to have fun with my friends and talk to everyone.

The Old You: I'm having a bad diet day because I got into a huge fight with my husband this morning. Carbs and sugar, here I come!

The New You: I'm still upset about fighting with my husband, but I'm not going to make it worse by eating sugar because food is not a Band-Aid. Shopping is another story, and maybe I'll treat myself to a new Dior eye shadow because that doesn't harm my health.

The Old You: Damn, I messed up so badly today with my food that tomorrow I will literally live on lettuce and water. I'll starve myself to make up for it.

The New You: There is no screwing up. Starving myself is not a good idea, because my body is a chemistry lab and not a bank account. If I made less-than-great choices on Friday, it doesn't mean I should starve on Saturday. Starving myself won't make me lose weight, but it will make me tired and lacking energy to do anything positive like working out. I will just start tomorrow with a healthful breakfast and get over it!

Don't Slip Down a Slippery Slope

Slips shouldn't be a daily event or carry on into the next day. If you feel as if you've had a night of slipping (and everyone has some of those), you should reach for a lifeline. That might be a close friend who is also on the plan and can talk to you about getting back on the horse. It's great to have a trainer or what I call "an accountability partner" to get your mind into the right place again.

This is certainly the time to get out your journal and revisit your goals. Don't rush through this process. Take the time to really think about it, so you can see it and then achieve it.

armed and dangerous

Rehearse a situation before you go into it. As a speaker, I do a lot of rehearsing because I want a certain outcome and I want to head off any and all problems. It's the same when you're going into a high-risk eating situation. Think about how you want the situation to go. Say to yourself, "I know when I get to a party I'm not going to touch the appetizers. I will have a drink in one hand and my purse in the other." Now you've got the details down and set yourself up to succeed!

How to Celebrate Your Success

People look at success as a number on the scale. I want you to reframe your thinking: you are successful if you did your workout for the day, made the right choices with your food, got a good night's sleep, and did your best to limit your stress. Each of these steps is making this a win-win situation for you. Now stop for a minute and celebrate all of the great things you're doing to succeed. I promise you that it will all come together over time and bring you the results you are looking for and deserve!

Instead of celebrating the ultimate outcome—which will come—be happy in the knowledge that you're doing the things you need in order to have those great arms. Celebrate the fact that you lifted 10 pounds a few days ago and 15 pounds today. Rejoice that you're now going to bed at 10 P.M. instead of midnight. Give yourself a pat on the back because you're eating a healthy breakfast now instead of grabbing a cup of coffee and bolting out the door. Feel good about the fact that you have your motivational picture right there in your purse as a safety blanket and security line.

Grab your journal and look at your progress. But be careful here, and please read on.

When Do I Weigh Myself?

The answer is once a week and on the same day each week. Keep track of your progress in your journal. Remember that you really must look at your overall body composition when you're considering progress. By body composition, I mean not just at weight but what that weight is made up of. How much is fat, and how much is fat-free mass (everything else)? The easiest way to do this is with a bioimpedance scale. These are available now for home use and are fairly inexpensive. Many local gyms also do body composition testing. Ideally you will record your weight, body fat, and hip and waist measurements weekly to ensure that you are losing fat while building muscle. Remember, muscle weighs more than fat (and acts like your own personal pair of Spanx by holding everything in tighter), so your weight loss will appear slower if you are losing fat and adding muscle.

You want to lose fat because you don't want to be fluffy. Your goal is to be solid as a rock. By the way, one great indicator that you are losing belly fat is that your waist starts denting in. If you see less you in the waist area, take a moment and say, "Congrats." (The flip side is that if your waist never seems to dent in, you're not losing belly fat and need to step up your workouts and review your eating.)

> ## How to Measure Your Waist and Hips
>
> Measure your waist by placing a tape measure around your body at the level of the uppermost part of your hipbone; this is usually at the level of your belly button. Measure your hips by placing your feet together and then measuring the widest part of your hips/buttocks.

Women are generally great at beating themselves up if they don't see the scale move each week. Please make sure that you're monitoring correctly, and don't lie to yourself. It doesn't help if you move the scale to that one weird part of the bathroom where the floor isn't even so that you see a lower number and feel better. Don't fudge on the measurements. You want to be accurate to keep real track of your progress.

Don't Be a TOFI

There is a phenomenon called TOFI. These are women who are Thin on the Outside and Fat on the Inside. You are TOFI if you are in the normal range for your weight but high in your body fat percentage (i.e., 30 percent). If this is you, you may not need to lose weight at all; you just need to add muscle and burn off fat weight. You will see your body fat percentage and measurements shift dramatically, so be sure you are monitoring more than just weight.

People Who Try to Throw You Off Track

You're doing fabulously on your program, and your willpower to succeed is made of steel. You are up in the morning, feeling great from your rejuvenating night of sleep, working out, bursting your heart out, and then doing your arm exercises with gusto and intensity. Your eating program is as close to perfect as possible.

Now you have to watch out for a hidden glitch: *other people who try to sabotage your success.* They are mostly food pushers who shove a brownie your way or even your significant other, who rolls over on a Sunday morning and says, "Blow off your exercise today and let's just hang out. I don't want you to get too muscular." (You can remind him until you turn green that women can't bulk up like that, but he's not really listening.)

Weight loss and a significant romantic partner can be a tricky thing. I lost a client who got so strong and lean (arms, legs, tummy, everything) that her newfound confidence in her body melded into the rest of her life. She became sure of herself in all areas of life as she became physically fit and quite the knockout.

Sadly, her husband was so afraid that she would leave him that he told her she was spending too much time focusing on working out. Then he started to bring home pizzas for dinner and suggested that they share high-calorie meals for "fun." This couple really needed to have a talk about what her new strength could mean to their relationship in a positive way.

A male client of mine was having great success on my program. He became thinner, stronger, and more confident as the weight came off and his muscle tone improved. His wife got very nervous about the new hunk sleeping next to her and started bringing him pieces of pie in bed.

It's scary to have a partner whom we love change quite a lot because we may wonder if the person will want to make other life changes, including dumping the status quo on the next pillow and finding a new partner.

Research shows that we tend to hang out with people who are similar to us in many ways, including income and body type. When one person in that group, or your mate, makes a major change, it can shine a light on you. It can become a case of why don't you do this too? If everyone in your group is failing at having a healthy body, you're all in the same boat. If one person succeeds and starts to look amazing, everyone else gets a little nervous after the initial "Oh, you look so great. What are you doing?"

The solution is simple. You may have to sit down with your

special people and have a talk with them about their dreams. You might have to set some boundaries in relationships and explain to everyone that it's not acceptable to bring home a pizza for dinner now or to bring a slice of pie (or any food, for that matter) to bed. It's just as easy to go out to a restaurant, where everyone can order according to his or her own diet plan. An Italian restaurant is a good choice because you can have delicious fish with fresh herbs, veggies, and a salad while the other people in your party have pasta and meatballs. You're 100 percent in charge of your own destiny.

What if the food pushers in your life just won't stop? You can say a firm no, but sometimes even that doesn't work. Perhaps it's your aunt who is the dessert pusher. She won't touch the dessert but wants to see you eat that concoction she made almost as if your eating that thick slice of chocolate pie is a way of living vicariously through you.

My advice is to simply say, "Gosh, that looks so awesome, Aunt Mary, but I'm just stuffed. Can I take a piece home for later?" And you know where that piece goes, right? Into a trash can. If you walk into the house with it, you're eventually going to go to bed with it and a cold glass of milk. Or simply tell your food pusher, "My stomach is feeling a little funky. I'll have to take a pass right now." It takes guts for someone to continue to push food on you when you've stated that you don't feel good. (Okay, it's a little white lie, but it protects everyone's feelings, including those of your mother, who is like a drug dealer with her apple pie surprise.)

Remember, you're a grown-up who is in control of what she eats, and no one can force-feed you unless they throw you to the ground and torture you. It's about learning how to set boundaries and about being in control. If you were at a party and someone said, "Hey, you have to do this heroin," would you do it? You wouldn't say to yourself, "You know what, I don't want to hurt her feelings, so I'll take a little hit off that crack pipe." Think of food as your drug. Someone is asking you to do something you don't want to, and you're fretting about not hurting his or her feelings. What about your feelings? What about your body? What about your health? Maybe this "food pusher" is wrapped up in food as love, but for you food is not love. It's no different than if it were a hard drug.

Don't Blow It: Exercise Now

We've focused a lot in this chapter about great eating habits, but I also want to take a moment and talk about your exercise plan. You're several weeks into the plan now, and you're still scheduling in exercise. You don't think about when and if you can fit your workout in but rather *when* you will absolutely be able to follow through with your commitment.

Women with great guns don't take consecutive days off from

exercising. You will schedule one day off each week, but no more. I always tell people to schedule six days a week to work out, and then if they fall short one day, it's not a criminal offense. It shouldn't happen, but it might every now and then if you're busy. The only other reason to take time off is when you're hurting or sick.

If you are feeling totally unmotivated, it's time to crank the tunes and tell yourself that you will at least do a miniworkout. Guess what, nine times out of ten you will get motivated once you get started. So pull out that motivational photo, unleash the tunes, and get moving.

7. Show 'Em

You've reached a turning point in your life, and it's a bit mind-boggling. Suddenly, after six weeks with me, you can enjoy your constitutional rights with a twist. Yes, *you* have the right to bare arms. Go ahead and flash your new arms in sleeveless dresses and cute tank tops while you're out among other people. I don't care if it's 32 degrees outside. You're going to want to show 'em in that beautiful cap-sleeve shirt. I don't care if you wear it to the grocery store. Just wear it proudly!

Ladies, we have one last lesson, and it revolves around vanity and your other right: *the right to look gorgeous and sexy.*

It's time for a little commercial break. Perhaps your arms haven't seen sunlight or experienced a cool breeze for more than a decade or two. Yes, you want to take your arms out for a test run, but there are matters of beauty to consider. Your arms may need a little more TLC—exfoliating, moisturizing, and even a little bronzer to really throw things over the edge. And please, I beg you: shave your armpits. This might seem like simple advice, but many of you haven't had to worry about this region coming into contact with other mortals for a long time.

In this chapter, I'll offer you special ways to show off the results of your hard work with a little help from some wonderful beauty gurus I call my Style Team. It's time to preen and pamper your arms a bit before you hit the red-carpet events in your life or even a PTA meeting. It's important to learn from the experts what type of clothing is perfect for arms of all shapes and sizes (and during your transition stages), plus some wonderful cosmetic tricks to make your arms look even smaller and aglow. I even asked my favorite photographer to offer crucial tips on how to pose for pictures so you can love how your arms are preserved for the ages in the family photo album.

Get ready to take your arms among the masses and wave them proudly! You got 'em; now flaunt 'em!

How Great Arms Will Revolutionize Your Life (Pass It On)

- Getting dressed in the morning will take a fraction of the time. All of your tops will look great. Close your eyes and just pick one.

- No more hours will be spent picking the right black T-shirt at the mall. You can actually wear colors now and will need only one or two great black tees. You'll save money on clothing because you won't be on the "hunt" for skinny-arm shirts. All shirts will be toned-and-sexy-arm shirts!

- You won't cringe when the summer halters and tanks hit the racks. Buy a few cute ones, and marvel at how great the fresh air feels on your skin.

- You'll finally be able to wear an adorable strappy sundress in the heat of the summer and not drag one of those cumbersome cover-ups with you. Shrug off your shrug for good.

- Bathing suit season won't be the trauma of the past. Have suit, will travel—to the beach. It's fun to wake up on a hot summer day and look forward to hitting the pool or beach with your loved ones.

- If you're going dancing with a significant other, you'll be able to wear a slinky dress. What feels better than skin-on-skin contact while you sway to beautiful music? It's much better than skin-on-shawl contact.

- You will feel more confident about having photos taken and not worry about looking like a linebacker because you're so wide across the top.

- You'll sleep better and handle stress with much more ease. Those two "side effects" of having gone through this program will affect your health positively in ways too numerous to list.

- You'll enjoy better stamina and energy in all activities. That includes having a better sex life. You're welcome!

- You'll feel much better about yourself, period. When you feel better about your body and have more energy because you're eating right and working out, that confidence will seep through to other areas of your life. Way to go!

Make Up Your Arms with Expert Carol Shaw

After weeks of toning and sculpting your arms, I want you to debut them with confidence and style. The Hollywood elite you see on the red carpet always put a little something extra on their arms to make them look even leaner and lovelier. I know the best person to turn to when it comes to getting your skin in great condition. Meet Carol Shaw, known internationally as the Red Carpet Authority, an amazing celebrity makeup artist and creator of the fantastic LORAC Cosmetics.

Carol, my ladies have been working extra hard to sculpt and tone their arms. Can you please give us your number-one tip for having gorgeous, sexy skin when it comes to our arms?

Do what the movie stars do, and rely on the magic of makeup! You can turn blah arms into supermodel arms. Yes, put a little makeup on your arms—all over your arms—and you will love the way they look. Any darker makeup bronzer or tan-colored makeup will help your arms appear slimmer. You can create the illusion of slimmer arms by just darkening your skin tone a bit. Take a big powder brush and just brush a powder foundation or bronzer on your arms.

How bold should you go?

Go a few shades darker—maybe one or two. You don't want to go so dark that it looks different from the rest of your body. I have a popular body product that's a body-bronzing luminizer with a little pearl in it. It has a light-reflecting ingredient that gives your skin a beautiful sheen.

Some stars like to contour their arms with makeup. Is this necessary?

Please don't get into contouring, where you use the makeup on just certain parts of your arms. No one can do this all by herself, and doing it the wrong way won't look natural. Just take the bronzer or makeup and cover your entire arm, up through your shoulder, and sweep up your neck. Your goal is not to go too dark or too light. You just want a beautiful, warm, tan, bronze glow that gives the illusion that your arms are thinner and longer. I love my own TANtilizer Award Show Glow product. It's a firming body-bronzing mousse. It's long-wearing and not a self-tanner, so there is no orange hue. It also helps the skin appear firmer and smoother while giving you a beautiful glow.

But please don't get this on your new white tank top, right?

Right. An additional tip is to let your arms dry before you put your clothes on, so nothing is stained. Also, make sure to wash your hands to get rid of excess product before you touch your clothing.

After a long winter, many women's arms look as though they're covered in bumpy white chicken skin. Can you exfoliate arms?

Nothing is worse than chicken skin! If you have rough arm skin, there's nothing wrong with exfoliating with any of the products you love. Just make sure to moisturize afterward. You should do this before putting on the bronzing makeup, because after you exfoliate and moisturize, the other products will just glide on.

Any other tips?

Remember that you're using the bronzer or makeup on your arms to even out your skin tone and work on luminosity. Your goal is to make your new arms look luscious, touchable, and sexy. And remember that darkening your skin with makeup will make your arms look even slimmer. Makeup will also enhance and help disguise things like little spots and moles.

Can we give a little bit of advice to our African-American and Hispanic ladies?

Any girl with a darker skin tone should use a great lotion on her arms and then cover it with a bit of darker bronzing powder. If you're really dark, use a lotion with some luminizer in it to give your arms a nice glow.

armed and dangerous

Do you have rough elbows that look almost white because the skin is so callused? Not pretty! Just gritty! Here's a great do-it-yourself home remedy that will gets rid of that dead skin. Cut a grapefruit in half and put both halves on paper plates on your kitchen table. Now lean forward and stick one elbow into each grapefruit half. The acid in the grapefruit will exfoliate all of that dead skin. Do this for ten minutes; then gently remove the rest of the dead skin with a loofah. Remember to moisturize.

Foods That Make Your Skin Glow

What you put into your body is also important when it comes to having beautiful arms and skin tone. Consider trying the following for a gorgeous glow:

- **Flaxseed.** The omega-3s in this will help keep your skin healthy and protect it from redness, rough patches, and scaling.
- **Pomegranate.** Loaded with antioxidants, this fruit helps with antiaging and is even said to boost your collagen.
- **Leafy green veggies.** They contain lutein, which protects your skin from sun damage and also helps increase its elasticity.
- **Dark chocolate.** Don't go crazy here, but a *little* bit will give you polyphenols, which keep the skin soft, smooth, strong, and hydrated.

Glowing Arms with Skin Care Expert Barbara Salomone

The amazing Barbara Salomone is the founder and CEO of the skin care line Bioelements and a licensed esthetician whose learning centers train other estheticians and skin care pros how to do fabulous facials and the most perfect full-body skin care. "Too many people ignore the skin on their body and just focus on their faces," Barbara says. "It's about smoothing and hydrating *all* of your skin, including your new amazing arms."

We're here to get our ladies to take care of the skin on their arms. What are your thoughts on full-body skin care?
Arms are the new legs. We're covering our legs with tights but showing our arms year-round. You can barely watch any TV anchor and not see her in a sleeveless dress when it's ten below in New York. You have to treat your arms the way you treat your legs in summer when you're showing them. It will take just a few simple steps to have soft, glowing arms.

Barbara, give us an arm skin care routine.
In the shower, use a good loofah or a little rougher washcloth or plastic puff and exfoliate your arms. You don't necessarily need a product. You just need friction to rub off the dead skin. The

next most important thing to do is to use a good rich lotion when you step out of the shower. Don't just think that because it's your body, you will slap on the cheapest lotion you can find and use that lotion only if and when you remember. If you go for a cheap lotion, you will be getting more water than ingredients. That's how cosmetic companies can fill a big-size bottle with lotion and price it cheaply. It just has more water in it. Those products don't necessarily give you the smoothest skin. You want to treat your arms to products that mimic a great facial moisturizer, such as a good, high-quality body cream. I like creams because they tend to be richer. Don't be afraid of breakouts. Very few people have oily skin on their arms.

What about self-tanner?

Every few days, I use a moderate self-tanner. This is especially important if your skin lacks color, is pasty or pale, or doesn't have a glow. It doesn't mean you want orange, fake suntan arms. There are a lot of nice products with a small amount of self-tanner that you can find in the drugstore. They give the skin a little glow and a little color.

You mentioned that you need a great body moisturizer for your arms and there are so many choices. What is key here to finding the perfect product?

You don't want to use a solid oil like coconut oil. That's what will tend to clog pores, even on your arms. What I like to see in a body moisturizer is the same ingredients you would see in facial skin care products. I like my own Vitalization Body Cream. You basically want high-quality botanical oils and shea butter plus antioxidants like green tea. I love shea butter because it is so skin smoothing. Essential oils are always good. You're better off staying away from highly perfumed body creams and lotions. Go for things with more natural beneficial elements. Your arms will love it!

Gorgeous Arms with Photography Expert Lesley Bohm

I have so many clients who tell me that they cringe when they see themselves in photos. It's not that they hate their smile or are having a bad-hair day. They despise how their arms look in the photos and even feel as though they're bigger on top than their mates are. For advice, I went to my favorite photographer, Lesley Bohm, who has been shooting celebs in Hollywood for more than twenty years.

Lesley, I know ladies who avoid pictures because they hate their arms. After they've done my program, this will be a thing

of the past. **But as my ladies transition into gorgeous arms, do you have any advice on how to take pictures they will love?**

My number-one tip, ladies, is confidence. Take that picture feeling confident. Even if you're not so thrilled about a body part like arms, people won't have a clue you have a problem. So walk in happy and feel great in your clothes, no matter what size you are right now. A great photo comes from within. Confidence is the sexiest thing. Even if you're not ready with your arms, your confident smile is what will be dazzling in the photo. Your personality will shine, and no one but you will study your arms as you work JJ's program. Of course, soon you will love your arms in photos.

For the women who still have fear about their arms looking too big in photos, is there any special wardrobe that helps?

First, get out of the black. Color is what draws your eye away from the body part and makes you think, "What a great color." You can also use a scarf or an amazing necklace to draw the eye to another part. If you're not happy with your arms yet, I'd do a wrap or necklace in a lovely color. If you're standing in the shot, wear fabulous shoes. Of course, wear sleeves if your arms are a big issue.

Any suggestions on how to stand to make the arms appear smaller in photos?

Never, ever stand straight on in front of the camera. This will guarantee that you will look your widest. It's a much softer look for women to stand at an angle with one shoulder toward the camera. When I shoot women who have on jeans or pants, I'll tell them to put their hands loosely in their pockets. It relaxes the shoulders and gives you a great clavicle in the picture. With hands in pockets, lift your elbows a bit. This will give a nice athletic look that shows off your muscles. If you're not wearing pockets, then pretend that you are and put your hands at your sides and lift your elbows a bit as you stand at an angle. You just made your triceps and biceps look great.

What if you're sitting down in a pose?
Don't smash your arms against your body. Lift your arms an inch away from the body to accentuate your muscle tone. Even if you don't have great muscle tone yet, you're accentuating leanness and the longness of your arm. If you're sitting in a chair for a pose, lean one elbow forward and the other back. Remember to never keep your arms glued to your sides. You can be stick thin, but if you pose that way you'll still look big. Actresses know how to sit at an angle, lean forward a bit, and even hold one knee with an arm to make the arm look longer.

What if you must go sleeveless at a big event? Any tips on how to make the photos look good when you're showing your entire naked arms?
What always looks great is a lovely sleeveless dress that goes up a bit higher on the shoulder—and always opt for a thinner strap. Skip the shrug, because they look awful in pictures. I will do

a thin cardigan layer for ladies over forty. Remember that your shoulders are a sexy point and your collarbone is probably beautiful. Shoulders are also elegant. To take the photo, stand sideways with your weight on your back foot and point your toe at the camera. This will thin you out everywhere, and you'll look great.

Now, what if your guy wants a romantic photo of the two of you and you're worried about looking larger than him in the arm area?

If the guy is taller than you, he will cover you up in the photo. One great way to take a nice shot is to be in front of him or facing each other. Or put your shoulders into his chest and lean on him a bit. Don't smash your arms into him. Remember, hand on your hip, and leave a bit of space so your arm isn't now squashed to his side. Ask your guy to angle into you. Now push your shoulder into him at an angle. He can also put his arm around your arm and hide the part you don't like, but remind him not to squash you there. Use your man as your accomplice!

Okay, let's drift off arms for a second and hit your best general advice for taking a gorgeous photo.

For a great face shot, bring your chin out, not up. Before the photographer shoots, look at the toe of your shoes and then look right into the camera. Don't lift your head up too high. You don't want any lasting memories of your nostrils!

armed and dangerous

Here's another reason to keep sipping that yummy green tea: it's a natural antioxidant that makes your skin look great. Many women believe that this is just for your face, but that's not true. The skin on your entire body, including your arms, will take on a new glow. So start brewing another pot at your earliest convenience.

Dress Your New Arms with Style Expert Tamara Gold

When it comes to dressing for successful arms, all styles are not created equal! Should you go sleeveless or try one of those cap sleeves that seem to be multiplying in stores at the mall? Do arms look better in sleeves that are three-quarter-length or T-shirt style? Why are tight shirts bad but loose ones just as horrible? It's all so confounding that naturally I turned to my wardrobe style expert, Tamara Gold, who dresses the stars to look their best.

Women are confused when it comes to sleeve length. Can you give us a few general rules?

Whatever sleeve you decide to wear, the biggest rule is to make sure it does not hit the heaviest part of your arm. You don't want the sleeve to call attention to the biggest and thickest part of this area, because it will make it look even heavier. Another great tip is never to buy sleeves that are tight. Make sure your tops have a little movement and breathing room in the sleeves. It's always better to buy a size up so the arms fit and then have the body altered by a great tailor for a perfect fit. Your tailor is your friend and secret weapon!

Shouldn't women also be careful not to wear tops that are too baggy?

Absolutely. Your shirts should have shape and form. Never go for boxy or baggy, because it will make this area look huge.

Any tricks if you don't want to go sleeveless?

I love a longer-sleeved arm that has a little slit up the side of it for fluidity. It still covers, but now it's interesting and sexy. You can wear a lighter fabric that moves for that same fluidity in the sleeve. But stay away from see-through sleeves, which don't look good on most people.

Where do you stand on the shrug?

If you have a great dress that's sleeveless, wear a cool scarf that wraps around your arms. Leave the top of your shoulders exposed. You're still dressed up and going sleeveless. But what you're showing is the top of your shoulders, which is a beautiful area on most women. You still get that feeling of a sundress.

Shrugs are fine, although some hit the wrong spot. I can never stand shrugs that are tight in the arms or too short. Make sure the shrug moves and isn't glued to your body. Not all shrugs are good shrugs. The key is to leave enough spare fabric so it's not completely tight and makes your arms look bigger.

What is a great sleeve length for most women?

I love three-quarter-length sleeves. You can fold them up a bit higher for a nice, casual look. You can dress them up for a fancy occasion or buy them with a little detail like a diamond or a little jewel on the sleeve. Beautiful trim makes these gorgeous, plus they will look good on arms that are a work in progress. You're not drawing attention to a part you don't like in these shirts.

What if you're forced against your will to wear a bridesmaid dress that's sleeveless? Is there something that can make even the most arm-phobic feel better?

Go to a great vintage store and buy a lovely shawl. Don't wear a jacket, because that will look too hard over a dress. A gorgeous shawl will add to the dress and not look like a shrug.

What about color and shirts?

Black is more slimming, but it also drains the color from your face. I'd suggest finding other neutral colors or a color that gives you the same feeling of slimming. But not black. Don't go too bright, but find a neutral that compliments your skin tone, eyes, and hair. Choose a color that makes you feel beautiful. Too many black shirts become a uniform. In many cases, skin goes sallow in winter and black really won't work for you. You can have a professional stylist do your color range if you really want to know what colors look great on you. It's great to wear colors that resonate with your skin tone. People will feel closer to you when they're talking to you if you wear those colors. Don't ever go for color-blocking sleeves. They only draw attention to your arms. The shirt and sleeve should be the same color.

Where do you stand on the cap sleeve, which is everywhere now?

The cap sleeve is the hardest one to wear. Yes, it's a great shirt for waiflike women. But the cap should be avoided unless you're very thin. It grabs you right in your fat. If you're toned, you can do cap, tanks, and halters. These shirts are best for women who have toned arms and gracefully elegant bone structure. If you're not that woman, thinner tank straps are actually better for you than thick tank straps that hit right under the arm.

So it really comes down to the individual.

Exactly. For me, the bell sleeve is great and I like long sleeves. The way they hit my hands and arms makes them perfect for me.

Tiny shoulder pads are fine if someone has very tiny shoulders, but if you're larger, forget it. Just remember that the worst is a fitted shirt that clings to you and encases your arms like sausages. Give your new arms a little breathing room, and you will look lovely!

A Final Word

I'm so proud of you for completing this program, but in actuality, it's only the beginning. You think I'm done with you in six weeks? Hardly! We're just beginning what I hope will be a long relationship, and soon I will have more books and videos to explore various paths to great health and fitness. Check out new developments, exciting products, my blog, my favorite burst trainer, additional arm exercises, and nutritional tips at my website, www .jjvirgin.com.

I made a promise early in this book that I would ask you to do only what was necessary to achieve dream arms. What's necessary now is that you stick to your program of smarter eating, arm exercises, cardio blasting, proper sleeping, and antistressing. Don't slip into old patterns and let these things slide. Practice them every single day. It's not just your arms that are benefiting here but your entire, much slimmer, more energetic, sexier body. I hope that doing all the above leads to a more confident you!

Above all, I wish you the best of health. I would love it if you would drop me a line when you get a chance and fill me in on your progress.

Until next time,

JJ

Appendix

JJ's Favorite Workout Music

- "Tears Dry on Their Own"—Amy Winehouse
- "Rock Steady"—Aretha Franklin
- "Ringa Ringa"—A. R. Rahman, Alka Yagnik (from *Slumdog Millionaire*)
- "Cradle of Love"—Billy Idol
- "Mony Mony"—Billy Idol
- "(Shine Your) Love Light Hope"—Bob Mould
- "Livin' on a Prayer"—Bon Jovi
- "I Don't Know Why I Love You"—The Brand New Heavies
- "Gimme More"—Britney Spears
- "Toxic"—Britney Spears
- "Womanizer"—Britney Spears

- "Dancing in the Dark"—Bruce Springsteen
- "Gonna Make You Sweat (Everybody Dance Now)"—C & C Music Factory
- "Wherever You Will Go"—The Calling
- "Love Has Fallen on Me"—Chaka Khan
- "Block Rockin' Beats"—The Chemical Brothers
- "Brio"—Chris Spheeris and Anthony Mazzella
- "A Whisper"—Coldplay
- "How Would You Feel"—David Morales
- "Just Another Love Song"—The Dead 60s
- "Riot Radio"—The Dead 60s
- "Savana Dance"—Deep Forest
- "Silence"—Delerium (featuring Sarah McLachlan)
- "Days Go By"—Dirty Vegas
- "Fall Behind Me"—The Donnas
- "Catch the Sun"—The Doves
- "Mercy"—Duffy
- "Stutter"—Elastica
- "Unbelievable"—EMF
- "Bring Me to Life"—Evanescense
- "Fergalicious"—Fergie
- "Paralyzer"—Finger Eleven
- "Big Love"—Fleetwood Mac
- "Generator"—Foo Fighters
- "How to Save a Life"—The Fray

- "Hammering in my Head"—Garbage
- "Gone Daddy Gone"—Gnarls Barkley
- "The Groove Line"—Heat Wave
- "I Like You So Much Better When You're Naked"—Ida Maria
- "Gravity"—James Brown
- "Don't Want to Fall in Love"—Jane Child
- "Rhythm Nation"—Janet Jackson
- "Switch"—Jazmine Sullivan
- "Are You Gonna Be My Girl"—Jet
- "Cold Hard Bitch"—Jet
- "Instant Karma"—John Lennon
- "I've Been Everywhere"—Johnny Cash
- "Any Way You Want It"—Journey
- "Stone in Love"—Journey
- "Sexy Back"—Justin Timberlake
- "Black Horse and the Cherry Tree"—K. T. Tunstall
- "Stand Up and Be Strong"—Keb' Mo'
- "Let It Rock"—Kevin Rudolf
- "Mr. Brightside"—The Killers
- "Jungle Boogie"—Kool and the Gang
- "Steal My Sunshine"—Len
- "Like a Prayer" (remix)—Madhouse
- "4 Minutes"—Madonna (featuring Justin Timberlake)
- "Amazing"—Madonna

- "Music"—Madonna
- "Ray of Light"—Madonna
- "Vogue"—Madonna
- "Fly Away" (Butterfly Reprise)—Mariah Carey
- "I'm That Chick"—Mariah Carey
- "Make It Happen"—Mariah Carey
- "Valerie"—Mark Ronson (featuring Amy Winehouse)
- "Got to Give It Up" (Part I)—Marvin Gaye
- "Billie Jean"—Michael Jackson
- "Black and White"—Michael Jackson
- "James Bond Theme"—Moby
- "Teenagers"—My Chemical Romance
- "Hot in Here"—Nelly
- "Perfect Kiss"—New Order
- "Hey Baby"—No Doubt
- "It's My Life"—No Doubt
- "Let's Get Physical"—Olivia Newton-John
- "The Saint"—Orbital
- "Blue Monday"—Orgy
- "Shake Ya' Tailfeather"—P. Diddy, Murphy Lee, Nelly
- "Feel Good Time"—Pink
- "God Is a DJ"—Pink
- "Trouble"—Pink
- "History Repeating"—Propellerheads

- "Spybreak!" (Short One)—Propellerheads
- "Take California"—Propellerheads
- "Don't Cha' "—Pussycat Dolls
- "When I Grow Up"—Pussycat Dolls
- "Ready to Go"—Republica
- "Don't Stop the Music"—Rihanna
- "Pon de Replay"—Rihanna
- "SOS"—Rihanna
- "Clubbed to Death"—Rob
- "Children"—Robert Miles
- "Fable"—Robert Miles
- "Pump Up the Jam"—Salt 'N Pepa
- "Future Love Paradise"—Seal
- "Loaded"—Seal
- "Waiting for You"—Seal
- "I'll Take You There"—Sean Paul
- "Back to Life"—Soul II Soul
- "Jungle Love"—Steve Miller Band
- "Gotta' Have You"—Stevie Wonder
- "Uptight"—Stevie Wonder
- "Desert Rose"—Sting
- "The Ballroom Blitz"—Sweet
- "You Make Me Feel (Mighty Real)"—Sylvester
- "You Wreck Me"—Tom Petty

- "Elevation"—U2
- "Where the Streets Have No Name"—U2
- "Ride"—The Vines
- "It's Raining Men"—The Weather Girls
- "Prickly Thorn but Sweetly Worn"—The White Stripes

Resources

Professional-Grade Supplements and Customized Nutrition

Metabolic Maintenance

www.Metabolicmaintenance.com

Metabolic Maintenance makes ThinSticks and ThinSticks Shakes. I use ThinSticks every day, and I have been amazed to find that my midmorning and midafternoon hunger pangs have completely vanished. ThinSticks are my secret weapon for overcoming weight loss resistance! This is the shake I personally formulated for Metabolic Maintenance to keep your appetite suppressed and your energy steady all day long.

JJ's Favorite Shakes

Essential Energy Packets, Essential Fiber, Paleobars, and my other favorite supplements

My team and I have spent years testing various supplements, shakes, fibers, and food bars to find a selection of products that taste great, offer superb nutritional benefits, and hold up to their promise of purity and quality. These are the very products I use personally and with my celebrity clients. They are available through select health care professionals and on my website store.

I recommend wild, cold-water fish as one of my favorite sources of protein and healthy fat. Vital Choice is a trusted source for fast home delivery of the world's finest wild Alaskan seafood and organic fare. Vital Choice captures the fresh-caught quality of fine, sustainably harvested Alaska Salmon and other Alaska and northwest Pacific seafood by processing and flash-freezing it within hours of harvest. It is then conveniently shipped to your door packed in dry ice to preserve its flavor and freshness. www.vitalchoice.com

General Nutrition Information

National Association of Nutrition Professionals

www.nanp.org

The NANP represents holistically trained nutrition professionals. Its mission is to enhance the integrity of the holistic nutrition profession through self-governance, educational standards, a rigorous code of ethics, and professional registration of holistic nutritionists. If you are a nutritionally oriented health care professional or interested in pursuing a career in this field, this organization is for you.

Emergen-C Packets and Shots

Available from Natural Partners

www.naturalpartners.com

Emergen-C is my favorite way to liven up water and sparkling mineral water. It contains 1,000 milligrams of vitamin C, B vitamins, electrolytes, and antioxidants that give you a natural boost of energy in a nutrient blast. And it tastes great. Try the raspberry, it's my current fave.

Fiber

Salba and Salba Rx

Salba

www.salba.com

Salba is "the world's most nutrient-dense functional food, combining two powerful ancient superfoods from Peru: salba and maca."

Dakota Gold Flax

Heintzman Farms

www.heintzmanfarms.com

This is my favorite flax—it is the Rolls-Royce of flaxseed. Once you try this, you will never go back! I order twelve bags at a time and store them in my fridge.

Exercise Equipment

X-iser

www.bursttoblastfat.com

Trash your treadmill—sprint on the X-iser! The days of 30- to 60-minute workouts on oversized machines are over. The sprint-training revolution is here. The science behind sprinting combined with the technology of the X-iser gives you a full cardio workout in just a few minutes a day. No, it is not just another stepper! The X-iser is specifically designed to allow any age and fitness level a way to sprint-train. No other stepping device can provide the same level of benefit.

Skin Care

Bioelements

www.bioelements.com

These are the skin care products I swear by, brought to you by one of the biggest names in the esthetics world, Barbara Salomone. Nothing shows off your arms like great skin, and Bioelements is your starting point!

LORAC

www.loraccosmetics.com

Carol Shaw, the founder of LORAC, is the Red-Carpet Authority for looking great. I rely on LORAC TANtalizer to make my arms look great even in the dead of winter ('cause guess what, you are going to want to go sleeveless no matter what the weather!). My photos were all taken with a healthy slathering of it!

Sleep Aids

Zeo Personal Sleep Coach

www.myzeo.com

The Zeo Personal Sleep Coach reveals how you *really* sleep and guides you in strategies to help you improve it. Because everyone's sleep pattern is different, Zeo combines your unique lifestyle and sleep data into a comprehensive program to help you get the sleep you need to feel your best. Zeo is composed of a comfortable wireless headband that tracks your sleep patterns and a bedside display to tell you about your deep sleep, REM sleep (when you dream), time to fall asleep, and other information. It also includes an email-based sleep-coaching service and an online account with tools to help you analyze trends in your sleep patterns.

Photography

Lesley Bohm

www.bohmphotography.com

Lesley is my go-to-gal for all photos. She can take you from good to great with a change of lighting or camera angles. People fly in from everywhere to work with Lesley, and if you need photos done, you will definitely want to visit her.

Stylist

Tamara Gold

http://theredlipstickreporter.com

Lesley and Tamara are my secret weapons for consistently great photos at every shoot. Plus, Tamara has amazing style tips in her Red Lipstick Reporter e-zine. Be sure to subscribe!

Scales

Tanita

www.jjvirgin.com/resources.html

Tanita scales are known worldwide for their quality, reliability, and accuracy. From the leaders in body composition comes a whole new level in measuring your competitive edge, Tanita's BC558 Segmental Body Composition Monitor. Why segmental? Simply put, segmental gives you more information than standard body composition monitors. This unique product gives individual body composition readings for each body segment: trunk, right arm, left arm, right leg, and left leg. The Ironman model BC558 is the one I recommend. Please use my code (jjvirgin) at checkout to get your free report "Understanding Body Composition." Just email your order number to info@jjvirgin.com, and we will send it to you right away.

Acknowledgments

I would like to thank the following people for their dedication and commitment to this book, to my vision, and to a healthier, sexier future for all.

My business manager and agent, David Dunham: thanks for tracking me down and then tenaciously pursuing me. I had been looking for someone who got it and me for years, and I am so fortunate to have your expertise, experience, and support.

My cowriter, Cindy Pearlman, for making this project a joy to do.

Jennifer Bergstrom, editor in chief at Simon & Schuster's Gallery Books, for making my dream a reality.

My editor, Patrick Price. I loved you the first time I met you.

You got it, you got me, and I knew you were the perfect person to edit this book.

Ali Brown and my Diamond mastermind group—Alexis Martin Neely, Lisa Sasevich, Sherie McConnell, Ciara Daykin, Michele DeKinder-Smith, Stacey Johnes and Regina Novickis, Karen Knowler, Kendall Summerhawk, and our token dude, Michael Reese—for being my kick in the butt, for holding me accountable, and for pushing me forward to bigger and better things. Oh, and the skinny-dipping in Maui worked wonders too.

Suzanne Somers for being such a wonderful role model and spokesperson for antiaging, health, and beauty. She is paving the way for all of us in integrated and holistic health, and I applaud her and admire her. It is an honor to know her.

Dr. Phil McGraw, for giving me a chance and the opportunity to get my message out to millions.

My team: Julia Zaslow, Dawna Sherrell, Mary Ann Guillory, Susan Tafralis, and Brett Enclade, who are with me on this mission to expand our vision to inspire the world to be proactive about health. You are all amazing in your commitment, your drive, and your unique abilities. I am so blessed to work with all of you.

My VIP clients: you have taught me so much over the years, and I am honored to work with you.

The National Association of Nutrition Professionals: it is a pleasure to be the president of such a progressive, transformative group.

A special thanks to others who have been wonderfully supportive of my vision and career, including my amazing PR team, Stacey Johnes and Regina Novickis; Tye and Dianna Smith of Natural Partners; Dr. Fabrizio Mancini and the faculty at Parker College; and my style team, Carol Shaw, Tamara Gold, Barbara Salomone, and Lesley Bohm.

My wonderful sons, Grant and Bryce, for bringing the fun factor into my life and for always keeping me on my toes. You bring balance into my life and a great perspective from the "other side."

And finally, my mom for always telling me I could be anything I chose to be. See, Mom, I do listen to you!

About the Author

JJ VIRGIN has successfully coached Hollywood elite, rock stars, heavyweight boxing champions, Olympians, and CEOs into shape using her powerful weight loss program. She is an on-camera nutrition and fitness expert, writer, professional speaker, spokesperson, and radio personality on nationally syndicated shows, including two seasons as the nutrition expert on *Dr. Phil*. A twenty-five-year board-certified veteran of the health and fitness industry, she lives in Palm Desert, California.